100
Short Cases
for the
MRCP

100
Short Cases
for the
MRCP

K. Gupta
MB, MRCP

Department of Medicine
Division of Gerontology and Geriatric Medicine
New York Medical College

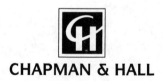

CHAPMAN & HALL

London · Glasgow · New York · Tokyo · Melbourne · Madras

Published by Chapman & Hall, 2–6 Boundary Row, London SE1 8HN

Chapman & Hall, 2–6 Boundary Row, London SE1 8HN, UK

Chapman & Hall, 29 West 35th Street, New York NY10001, USA

Chapman & Hall Japan, Thomson Publishing Japan, Hirakawacho Nemoto Building, 7F, 1-7-11 Hirakawa-cho, Chiyoda-ku, Tokyo 102, Japan

Chapman & Hall Australia, Thomas Nelson Australia, 102 Dodds Street, South Melbourne, Victoria 3205, Australia

Chapman & Hall India, R. Seshadri, 32 Second Main Road, CIT East, Madras 600 035, India

First edition 1983
Reprinted 1984, 1986, 1987, 1991

© 1983 K. Gupta

Printed in Great Britain by Ipswich Book Co., Ipswich

ISBN 0 412 25230 9

A catalogue record for this book is available from the British Library

Library of Congress Cataloging-in-Publication data

Gupta, K.
  100 short cases for the MRCP.

  Includes index
  1. Physical diagnosis — Case studies. I. Title II. Title: One hundred short cases for the MRCP.
RC76.G86 1983 616.07'54'0926 82–23477
ISBN 0–412–25230–9

Contents

SECTION 2. CARDIOVASCULAR SYSTEM

SECTION 3. RESPIRATORY SYSTEM

SECTION 4. ABDOMEN

SECTION 5. CENTRAL NERVOUS SYSTEM

SECTION 6. LOOKING AT THE FUNDI

SECTION 7. LOOKING AT THE HANDS

SECTION 8. LOOKING AT THE LEGS

SECTION 9. DERMATOLOGY

Foreword

The purpose of the clinical part of the examination for the membership diploma of the Royal College of Physicians (UK) is to ensure that successful candidates have acquired a high standard of history taking and physical examination, and are capable of sound judgement in interpreting their findings, in advancing sensible differential diagnoses and in planning investigations and management, taking into consideration all physical, psychological and social factors. The achievement of this high standard depends greatly on the depth and breadth of the candidate's experience at the bedside and in the clinic, and on the responsibility which he has held for making important clinical decisions under the general guidance of a senior physician. Experience of this kind sharpens the clinical acumen of the trainee physician and engenders in him a disciplined routine of physical examination which he can appropriately modify to deal with a wide spectrum of clinical patterns of disease. The presentation of 'short cases' in the clinical part of the MRCP examination specifically concentrates on this aspect of training.

   This little book is intended to heighten the candidate's awareness of commonly encountered clinical patterns of abnormal physical signs and to draw his attention to the kind of questions he should be repeatedly asking himself as the pattern unfolds before him. Hopefully, it will stimulate within him a freer association of ideas, which he can then proceed to test further as his physical examination proceeds. The book makes no attempt to be comprehensive. It understandably centres upon the more commonly encountered patterns of physical signs in clinical practice in the United Kingdom and upon a number of rarer conditions which have traditionally been selected for examinations because they present with striking physical signs. The aspiring candidate for the membership would do well to browse through this book and to annotate and expand upon it in ways related to his own personal experiences. He would also be well advised to ask a senior colleague to observe him in action when presented with a variety of 'short cases' and so discover whether he has learnt his lesson and developed a comprehensive, efficient and imaginative approach to each problem.

This book is clearly the product of an author who, together with his advisers, has been subjected to the rigours of the MRCP clinical examination, and I am confident that the advice contained herein will be of inestimable value to those who follow in his footsteps.

J.M. Ledingham
MD, FRCP
Emeritus Professor of Medicine

Preface

By the time a candidate sits for Part II of the MRCP examination, he or she will have acquired a good theoretical knowledge of medicine, along with practical experience of dealing with a significant number of patients while working as a junior hospital doctor. Most British medical examinations for higher diplomas, in particular the MRCP, are well known for the considerable importance they attach to the clinical section of the examination: to fail this part of the examination is to fail the whole examination. Most candidates find the 'short cases' more difficult to pass compared with the 'long case', where the candidate has a full 60 minutes at his disposal. In a non-examination situation, such as day to day hospital practice, one is relatively at ease, with plenty of time to examine the patient, take a good history and at times to check and recheck the presence or absence of a particular heart murmur or hepatic or splenic enlargement. This is not the case under examination conditions, where the candidate is being watched constantly by two examiners and can be obsessed with fear of failure. Not surprisingly, this puts extra pressure on the candidate who is usually expected (without enquiring about the patient's symptoms) not only to carry out the physical examination in an established fashion, but to correlate the relevant findings and present a short case report in a limited period of 3–5 minutes. In thirty minutes, the candidate is expected to examine as many as six to eight short cases. Speed and thoroughness in physical examination are vital in arriving at a sensible probable diagnosis.

This book is intended mainly to help final MRCP candidates, to develop a methodical, accurate and comprehensive approach to the commonly-given short cases so that they can avoid repeated half-hearted demonstrations of physical signs. Besides MRCP, this book should be of great help for qualifying examinations in medicine and other postgraduate qualifications that are equivalent to MRCP, such as FRACP (Australia and New Zealand), FCP (South Africa) and MD (India).

K. Gupta
MB, MRCP (UK)
The London Hospital, E1

Looking at the Patient

1. Paget's disease of the bone (skull)

You may be asked to look at the face.

Locally

- Look at the skull for enlarged calvarium.
- Palpate the scalp since the surface may be corrugated (irregular).
- Look for any evidence of loss of hearing due to 8th nerve involvement by Paget's disease.

Elsewhere

- Look for bowing of the legs.
- Look for signs of high output cardiac failure, e.g. a collapsing pulse, raised JVP, cardiomegaly, hepatomegaly and oedema of the legs.
- Look for deformities of other bones, e.g. pelvis, humerus, clavicles, etc.

Common questions

Q. What two important investigations would you ask for?
A. (i) X-ray of the skull.
   (ii) Serum calcium, phosphorus and alkaline phosphatase.
Q. What are the complications of Paget's disease?

A. (i) Bone pains.
  (ii) Pathological fractures.
  (iii) Cranial nerve palsy, most commonly of 8th nerve.
  (iv) Congestive cardiac failure.
  (v) Osteogenic sarcoma.

2. Acromegaly

You may be asked to look at the patient. Note the following features:

Locally

- Look carefully at the face – enlarged lips, accentuated skin folds with characteristic coarsening of the facial features.
- Look for prognathism (protrusion of the lower jaw).
- Look for any scar of operation on the skull.
- Always check for visual field defect, e.g. bitemporal hemianopia.

Elsewhere

- Look at the hands, which are unusually thick and fleshy.
- Shake hands with the patient and you may get the feeling of losing your hand in a mass of dough.

Discussion

Acromegaly results from the excessive secretion of human growth hormone, caused by an acidophilic adenoma of the pituitary, less commonly by a chromophobe adenoma and rarely by a histologically normal pituitary. Acromegaly is characterized by an increase in the size of the viscera, bones and soft tissue of the hands, feet, supraorbital ridges, sinuses and lower jaw (prognathism). Glycosuria occurs in about 30% of untreated cases and hypertension is not uncommon.

Common questions

Q. What three investigations will you ask for?
A. (i) X-ray skull (enlargement and erosion of sella turcica), hands (tufting of terminal phalanges), feet (heel pad thickness).
(ii) Serum growth hormone level (fasting levels in excess of 10 ng ml^{-1}).
(iii) Blood sugar.

Q. How can the condition present?
A. (i) Headaches and visual problems.
(ii) Paraesthesia of the hands and feet.
(iii) Change in size of the hat, ring or shoes.
(iv) Arthralgia and excessive sweating.
(v) Diabetes mellitus.
(vi) Hypertension.

3. Hydrocephalus

You may be asked to look at the skull or face of a patient with congenital hydrocephalus who has survived into adult life.

- Note that the skull is globular, smooth and symmetrically enlarged and the facial bones are normal.
- Both eyeballs are prominent (mild to moderate exophthalmos) and are rather pushed downwards so that the upper part of the sclera is visible.
- Look for signs of raised intracranial pressure, e.g. fundi for papilloedema or optic atrophy. Very often patients with 'normal pressure' hydrocephalus appear in such examinations.

Common question

Q. What is the differential diagnosis?
A. (i) Paget's disease of the skull. In these patients the skull is irregularly enlarged and there may be bowing of the tibia as well.
(ii) Achondroplasia. In this autosomal dominant disorder,

the person is carrying a normal size skull with a short stature and thus the head appears to be enlarged in relation to the height.

4. Hyperthyroidism

You are likely to be asked to look at the face.

Locally

- Look carefully at the prominent eyeballs (exophthalmos) and describe whether symmetrical on both sides or not.
- Look for lid retraction (visible sclera with staring look and wide palpebral fissure and lid lag (delayed movement of the upper eyelid).
- Check the movements of the eyeball in all directions for any external ophthalmoplegia and ask the patient about double vision.
- Look for any thyroid enlargement – the size and the surface of the gland.
- Ask the patient to swallow sips of water and see if the swelling in the neck moves with deglutition (this confirms that the swelling is of thyroid gland, since the thyroid gland is ensheathed by the pretracheal fascia).
- Palpate the gland for any nodules and the consistency.
- Auscultate for any bruit over the gland.

Elsewhere

- Ask the patient to spread the fingers of both hands and look for fine tremor and clubbing (acropachy).
- Feel the pulse (radial) for any tachycardia or irregularity.
- Look at the shins for pretibial myxoedema.
- Examine shoulder girdle for wasting (thyrotoxic myopathy).

Discussion

Hyperthyroidism occurs much more frequently in women than in men (8:1), usually in early adult life, and is commonly used both as a 'short' and 'long' case. Various investigations and the interpretation of thyroid function tests, treatment of the condition (indications for drug treatment), radioiodine therapy and surgery should be remembered.

Common questions

Q. What is T_3 thyrotoxicosis?

A. This is a form of thyrotoxicosis, where the patients have normal levels of plasma T_4 (thyroxine), but raised T_3 (triiodothyronine) levels. The clinical features are exactly as those of T_4 excess.

Q. Tell me something about the aetiology of Graves' disease.

A. The exact aetiology remains unclear, but it is thought to be an autoimmune condition. At one time an antibody, long-acting thyroid stimulator (LATS), was considered to be responsible. Now LATS has been disregarded as a major cause of Graves' disease, since it is not present in all patients with Graves' disease and its levels do not correlate with the presence or severity of the eye signs. Another antibody – human specific thyroid stimulator (HTS) has been blamed in the past. Although not certain, Graves' disease is now considered to be attributable to an antibody to the TSH-receptor.

Q. What is lid lag?

A. Lid lag results when the sclera between the upper lid and cornea becomes visible as the patient is asked to follow the finger downwards from the position of maximum elevation.

Q. What is pretibial myxoedema?

A. Localized myxoedema, appearing as thickened raised plaques with a peau d'orange appearance over the dorsum of the legs or feet, in untreated or treated cases of hyperthyroidism, is called pretibial myxoedema. Clubbing of the fingers, toes or exophthalmos may also be seen (thyroid acropachy).

5. Hypothyroidism

You are likely to be asked to look at the face.

Locally

- Note the coarse features on the facies – dry thickened skin, puffiness around the eyelids.
- Note sparse hair over the scalp with loss of hair from outer third of the eyebrow. Do remember that this is not considered to be a very helpful sign for hypothyroidism nowadays.
- Ask the patient their address and note that the speech is slow, monotonous and often hoarse and croaking in character.

Elsewhere

- Slow pulse rate.
- Rough and dry skin of the hands.
- Demonstrate the slow relaxation of the ankle jerk.
- Look for any scar of previous operation or thyroid enlargement.
- Look for any evidence of carpal tunnel syndrome (see Case 83).

Discussion

The distinction between hypothyroidism and myxoedema is important because although all myxoedematous patients show diminished thyroid function, not all patients who are suffering from a lack of thyroid hormone show myxoedema and because of this the diagnosis of hypothyroidism is often overlooked. Swelling due to myxoedema never pits on pressure.

Common question

Q. What one question would you like to ask the patient?
A. Do you prefer cold or hot weather? Myxoedema patients prefer hot weather whereas thyrotoxic patients find cold weather much more pleasant.

6. Cushing's syndrome

You may be asked to look at the patient. Note the following features:

- 'Moon'-shaped rounded face with plethoric appearance.
- 'Buffalo hump' – prominent supraclavicular and dorsal cervical fat pads.
- Truncal obesity.
- Purple striae over the abdomen. Purpura and spontaneous bruising over the extremities.
- Acne and hirsutism.
- Note the blood pressure as patients are often hypertensive.

Discussion

Hypersecretion of glucocorticoids produces Cushing's syndrome. This is usually caused by bilateral adrenocortical hyperplasia due to an excess of pituitary adrenocorticotrophic hormone (ACTH). Less commonly it is caused by an adrenal adenoma or rarely by a carcinoma.

Common question

Q. What investigations do you want to do?
A. (i) Check for high level and loss of diurnal variation of plasma cortisol.
(ii) Urinary steroid measurements (urinary output of free cortisol is increased).
(iii) Dexamethasone suppression test. Small dose dexamethasone test is done to establish that the patient has hypercortisolism whereas the large dose dexamethasone test is used to determine whether the adrenal function is under pituitary control or not. Only in cases of excess ACTH production from the pituitary, is suppression of the adrenal function seen. Patients with adrenal tumour and ectopic ACTH syndrome fail to show significant suppression. Measurements of ACTH level help in such circumstances as ACTH is low in autonomous adrenal function but is raised in ectopic ACTH syndrome.

(iv) CXR and X-ray pituitary fossa.

(v) Abdominal ultrasound scanning.

(vi) CT scan for confirmation of adrenal tumour.

7. Achondroplasia

You may be asked to look at the patient.

• Note the small stature of the patient with gross shortening of all four limbs but with a normal trunk length.

• Note that the skull appears to be enlarged but this is in fact due to abnormally short stature of the person and not an actual enlargement of the skull.

• Note that the forehead is rather prominent and bulging with a depressed bridge of the nose.

• Ask the patient to stand and note some degree of dorsal kyphosis with compensatory posterior rotation of the sacrum and pelvis.

• Note that the hands are small with all fingers being almost of equal length.

Common questions

Q. What is the inheritance of this disorder?

A. Autosomal dominant.

Q. What is the differential diagnosis?

A. (i) Hydrocephalus.

(ii) Paget's disease of bone.

(iii) Rickets.

Q. Does the condition affect the intelligence of the patients?

A. No – they have normal intelligence.

8. Kleinfelter's syndrome (47 XXY)

You may be asked to look at the patient. Note the following features:

- A tall person with disproportionately long lower extremities.
- Gynaecomastia (present in about 50% of cases, therefore absence of gynaecomastia does not rule out the condition).
- Firm and small testes. This is because of the atrophy and hyalinization of the tubules.

Discussion

Clinical variation in Kleinfelter's syndrome is great and many males who appear to be normal and have normal intelligence are found to have the 47 XXY karyotype in the course of an investigation for infertility. As the number of Xs increases, the chances of mental retardation increases, e.g. patients with 48 XXYY, 48 XXXY, 49 XXXXY are invariably mentally retarded.

9. Mongolism

You may be asked to look at a child, or even a young adult, with mongolism.

- Note the small stature of the patient.
- Note that the skull is small and brachycephalic, and that the face is expressionless, and the patient appears to be mentally retarded.
- Note that the eyes are slanted and epicanthal folds are usually present. There may be a convergent squint and, in the first year of life, there may be Brushfield's spots seen around the periphery of the iris.
- Note that the bridge of the nose is flattened, and the tongue is rather large and protruding.
- Note that the hands are short and broad, with a single palmar crease ('Simian crease'), and the fingers are small; the little finger is incurved, with an ulnar convexity and with an absent second phalanx.
- Now examine the heart for any congenital heart disease, e.g. atrioventricular septal defects, which are present in up to 30% of mongols.

Common question

Q. What is the genetic abnormality in these patients?
A. In most cases, it is a trisomy of chromosome 21, i.e. these patients have 47 chromosomes instead of the normal 46. In some cases, it is due to mosaicism or translocation of the chromosomes.

10. Systemic lupus erythematosus

You may be asked to look at the face. Note the following features:

- An erythematous lesion over the bridge of the nose extending to both cheeks which looks like a butterfly.
- Look for area of scarring, telangiectasia, keratotic plugging, hypopigmentation (in the centre) and hyperpigmentation (at the edges) in the butterfly lesion.
- Look for alopecia over the scalp.
- In the hands look for evidence of arthropathy usually involving the metacarpophalangeal (MCP) and proximal interphalangeal (IP) joints. Ulnar deviation of the fingers and subluxation of the proximal IP joints may be seen without X-ray evidence of erosion.
- Look for evidence of pleurisy with or without pleural effusion.
- Look for pericardial rub and heart murmurs.

Discussion

Systemic lupus erythematosus is an inflammatory connective tissue disorder of unknown aetiology occurring predominantly in young women. Various systems of the body are affected and therefore the clinical features include: facial erythema, purpura, alopecia, photosensitivity, arthritis, pleuritis, pericarditis, renal involvement and psychosis.

Common questions

Q. What investigations would you ask for?
A. (i) Full blood count including platelet count and ESR.

(ii) Antinuclear factor, LE cells, DNA binding.
(iii) Urine for protein and casts.
(iv) Chest X-ray.

Q. What is discoid lupus?
A. It is a chronic skin condition characterized by erythematous lesions with excessive scaling, atrophy, scarring, hypo- and hyper-pigmentation. Lesions subside and leave deep scars behind the face, neck and arms. The scalp also may be involved. Only a few of these patients develop systemic lupus erythematosus. Conversely some patients with SLE may have discoid lesions.

Q. Name three drugs which cause SLE-like syndrome?
A. (i) Hydrazides (hydralazine and isoniazid).
   (ii) Phenytoin.
   (iii) Procainamide.

Q. Name three drugs which exacerbate SLE?
A. (i) Penicillin.
   (ii) Sulphonamides.
   (iii) Oral contraceptive.

11. Scleroderma (systemic sclerosis)

You may be asked to look at the patient. Note the following features:

Locally

- Thickened, taut and waxy skin with thin hairs on the face specially around the lips should give a high index of suspicion.
- Thickened skin over the fingers with disappearance of the normal skin folds over the knuckles. The joints of the fingers may be swollen as a result of polyarthralgia.
- Tiny areas of ulceration at the ends of the digits as a result of vasculitis.
- Areas of telangiectases on the face, lips, tongue and fingers. Subcutaneous calcification in the fingers is common.

Discussion

Scleroderma or progressive systemic sclerosis is a collagen disorder of unknown cause characterized by diffuse fibrosis and vascular abnormalities in the skin, joints, gastrointestinal tract, lung, heart and kidneys.

Common questions

Q. What investigations would you ask for?
A. (i) ESR, antinuclear factor.
   (ii) Chest X-ray (pulmonary fibrosis).
   (iii) Barium meal (dilated, atonic oesophagus).

Q. What is CRST syndrome?
A. Calcinosis of the skin, Raynaud's phenomenon, sclerodactyly and telangiectasia constitute CRST syndrome. Patients with CRST syndrome are thought to have an association with primary biliary cirrhosis.

Q. What is the prognosis of systemic sclerosis?
A. Most patients with systemic sclerosis die within 3–5 years after the diagnosis has been made. Patients with mainly skin changes usually have a better prognosis than those with visceral involvement. Also the condition is usually more severe in black females.

12. Lupus pernio

You may be asked to look at the face. Note the following features:

Locally

• A bluish discoloration on the nose.
• Look for any plaques, scars or keloids.
• Look for any evidence of uveitis.
• Look for any evidence of facial nerve palsy.

Elsewhere

- Look for the presence of erythema nodosum.
- Check for lymphadenopathy.
- Look for any swelling of the phalanges (bone cysts).

Common question

Q. What two investigations would you ask for?
A. (i) Chest X-ray (hilar lymphadenopathy, infiltration and fibrosis).
(ii) Kveim test.

Q. What is the significance of lupus pernio?
A. Sarcoidosis of the upper respiratory tract (more common in women) is associated with increased risk of developing lupus pernio and early use of steroids is advocated to prevent this disfiguring complication. Kveim test is almost always positive in patients with sarcoidosis of upper respiratory tract with lupus pernio.

13. Xanthelasma

You may be asked to look at the patient. Note the following features:

- Raised, yellow plaques about the eyelids near the inner canthus.
- Look for xanthomas elsewhere in the body, e.g. palms, knuckles, tendoachilles, etc.
- Look for jaundice (obstructive jaundice).
- Does the patient look myxoedematous?
- Does the patient have swelling of the eyelids and legs (nephrotic syndrome)?

Discussion

Deposits of lipids, predominantly cholesterol in the dermis or subcutaneous tissue around the eyelids are called xanthelasma.

Various conditions associated with a high serum cholesterol level should be remembered, e.g. familial hypercholesterolaemia, prolonged obstructive jaundice, myxoedema, nephrotic syndrome and diabetes mellitus. Not infrequently xanthelasma is seen in the presence of normal serum cholesterol level.

Common question

Q. What are the three main types of xanthomas?

A. (i) Eruptive xanthomas. These are seen as firm raised papules with pale yellow centres over the buttocks, elbows, knees and dorsum of the arms. Familial hypertriglyceridaemia, diabetes mellitus and/or alcohol consumption are common conditions for such xanthomas.

(ii) Planar or palmar xanthomas. These xanthomas are seen in the palmar and digital creases and are commonly seen in Type III hyperlipoproteinaemia.

(iii) Tendon xanthomas. These occur in extensor tendons at the back of the hands and the achilles or the patellar tendons. These are believed to be specific for familial hypercholesterolaemia.

Nb. Remember the Fredrickson's classification of hyperlipidaemia.

14. Hereditary haemorrhagic telangiectasia

You may be asked to look at the patient. Note the following features:

- Small flattened telangiectasic lesions on the lips, oral and nasal mucosa, tongue and the tips of fingers and toes.
- Patients are usually anaemic since the lesions tend to bleed spontaneously or as a result of trivial trauma.

Discussion

Hereditary haemorrhagic telangiectasia or Osler–Rendu–Weber syndrome is inherited as an autosomal dominant condition.

Bleeding from the superficial lesions may be profuse. Visceral telangiectasia or AV aneurysms may occur in the lungs, liver and spleen. Epistaxis and gastrointestinal bleeding is more common and much more serious. Blood transfusions are usually required for acute haemorrhages. Continuous iron therapy to correct the iron-deficiency anaemia is usually necessary for many patients. It is important to remember that small telangiectatic lesions may also be seen in scleroderma, but the character of the skin remains unchanged in hereditary haemorrhagic telangiectasia, whereas in scleroderma the skin becomes thick, taut and difficult to pinch.

Common question

Q. What is the role of hormones in the treatment?
A. Oestrogens are considered to be of value in the therapy and in many cases reduce epistaxis. Their mode of action is probably by causing squamous metaplasia of the nasal mucosa. In males, testosterone is also required to avoid undesirable feminizing effects.

15. Dermatomyositis

You may be asked to examine a patient whose main complaint may be weakness of proximal muscles.

- Look carefully for the presence of any skin rash over face, shoulders or the arms. 'Heliotrope' rash with suffusion of the eyelids may be diagnostic of this disorder.
- Look for any wasting of the proximal muscles, present only in the late stages.
- Test for the strength of these muscles. Weakness may be striking at the hips or shoulders.
- Look for any areas of muscle tenderness by palpating the various muscles.
- Note and demonstrate that the reflexes are depressed in the affected muscle groups, but there is no sensory deficit.
- Examine the lungs for any evidence of interstitial fibrosis or carcinoma.

- Examine the breasts and palpate the abdomen for any evidence of carcinoma (breast, stomach, uterus or ovary) which is seen in more than 50% of the cases.

Common question

Q. What five investigations would you ask for?
A. (i) Raised ESR and full blood count (leucocytosis).
(ii) Estimation of muscle enzymes (CPK and transaminases are raised).
(iii) Electromyography (fibrillations and polyphasic discharges).
(iv) Muscle biopsy (inflammation and necrosis).
(v) Barium swallaw (atonic dilated oesophagus).

16. Dystrophia myotonica

You may be asked to look at the patient. Note the following features:

- Look at the wasting of face and neck muscles, particularly the sternal head of sternomastoids.
- Look at the eyes very carefully for bilateral ptosis, which is quite commonly seen.
- Look for cataracts.
- Frontal balding is also commonly associated.
- The distal parts of the limbs may also show some muscle wasting, especially in the forearms. Check the grip of the hands on both sides and look for slow relaxation of the muscles.
- Testicular atrophy must be looked for as well.

Discussion

Both muscular dystrophy and myotonia are seen in this autosomally dominant condition which usually begins in adult life. Mental retardation may also be seen. There is no satisfactory treatment available, but phenytoin and steroids have been used for symptoms of myotonia.

17. Facioscapulohumeral muscular dystrophy

You may be asked to look at the patient.

- Look at the bilateral symmetrical weakness of facial and sternoclavicular muscles.
- Note bilateral ptosis without any over-action of the frontalis muscle.
- Examine and note the weakness of sternal head of the pectoral muscles.
- Ask the patient to push against a wall with the arms extended and note the winging of the scapulae.
- Also examine the muscles of the pelvic girdle and lower limbs as in later years they may also be involved.
- Demonstrate the loss or poverty of reflexes in the affected muscles with no sensory deficit.

Common questions

Q. What is the inheritance of this disorder of muscles?
A. Autosomal dominant.

Q. What are the two other important possible diagnoses?
A. (i) Dystrophia myotonica.
   (ii) Myasthenia gravis.

Q. Does it affect the life expectancy?
A. Not usually.

18. Ankylosing spondylitis

You may be asked to look at a patient or at the back as the patient is standing.

- Note the loss of normal lumbar concave curve (lordosis) which is due to the muscle spasm and involvement of adjacent spinal joints.
- Note the flexion deformity of the hips and neck, and see if the patient is walking in a stooped posture with stiff ankylosed spine and has difficulty in seeing ahead.

17

- Ask the patient to bend forward and notice the limitation of joint movements. The patient may bend over as if he has a board in his back. Similarly the lateral movements of the spine are limited.
- Measure the expansion of the chest and this may be affected due to costovertebral joint involvement. Vital capacity is reduced but vital capacity:forced expiratory volume remains normal.
- Check for the movements of neck and sacroiliac joints. These may be limited too.
- Listen to the heart for the murmur of aortic incompetence.
- Look for any evidence of uveitis.

Common question

Q. What three investigations would you like to do?
A. (i) Hb, ESR.
   (ii) Spine X-ray including sacroiliac joints.
   (iii) Chest X-ray (bilateral apical fibrosis).

19. Turner's syndrome

You may be asked to look at the patient.

- Short stature of the patient should make you suspicious of this condition.
- Look for webbing of the neck.
- Look for shield chest – broad chest with widely apart nipples and poorly developed breasts.
- Look for signs of coarctation of aorta as described in Case 36.
- Note the increased carrying angle of both elbows.
- Look for short fourth metacarpals.

Discussion

Turner's syndrome is the most common cause of primary ovarian failure. The chromosomal anomaly is the presence of only one X chromosome in all cells. A number of patients with Turner's syndrome are mosaics, e.g. 46 XX, 47 XXX; menstrual function and reproduction in a patient with Turner's phenotype must be due to this mosaicism.

Common question

Q. What single investigation would you ask for?
A. Cytogenetic analysis of buccal mucosa (absent chromatin bodies in most cases but mosaics are chromatin positive).

20. Laurence–Moon–Biedl syndrome

You may be asked to look at the patient.

- Note that the patient is obese and may also be a dwarf.
- Examine the hands and feet and look for polydactyly or syndactyly, or a scar of operation for separation of fingers or toes.
- Look for evidence of genital hypoplasia: poorly developed testis, penis and pubic hair in a male patient or poorly developed breasts in a female patient.
- Now examine the visual acuity, field of vision and fundi for features of retinitis pigmentosa, with or without optic atrophy.
- Note that the patient appears to be mentally retarded.

Common questions

Q. What is the inheritance of this disorder?
A. It is thought to be autosomal recessive.

Q. Where is the lesion in this syndrome?
A. Probably in the hypothalmus.

21. Parkinsonism

You may be asked to look at the patient. Note the following features:

- The patient is invariably elderly with an expressionless (mask-like) face.
- Note the pill rolling movements of the thumbs and the fingers on one or both sides. The tremor are coarse, slow, present at rest and disappear on voluntary movement.
- Check for the presence of other extrapyramidal signs such as cogwheel rigidity of the limbs.
- Test the glabellar tap sign (on repeated tapping of the glabella the Parkinsonian patient continues blinking), though this is not thought to be very reliable.
- Ask the patient to walk and note the short shuffling character of his gait with absence of normal swinging of the arms. On pushing the patient you may notice the festinating gait, wherein the patient is hurrying with small steps in a stooped posture as if trying to catch up with his own centre of gravity.

Discussion

Parkinsonism is characterized by slowness and poverty of emotional and voluntary movement, rigidity and tremor. Parkinson's disease itself is idiopathic, and is due to decreased dopamine content in axon terminals of cells projecting from the substantia nigra to the caudate nucleus and putamen. In Parkinson's disease the mental state remains normal and there are no upper motor neurone signs since the pyramidal tracts remain intact. Tremor or rigidity may occur alone or coexist.

Common questions

Q. What are the causes of Parkinsonism?
A. Idiopathic.
   Drug induced (phenothiazines).
   Postencephalitic.
   Toxic (copper in Wilson's disease; manganese or carbon monoxide poisoning).
   Arteriosclerotic.

Q. Are tremor helped by L-dopa.
A. No, L-dopa helps only the dyskynesia and sometimes the tremor may be worsened by L-dopa.

22. Choreiform movements

You may be asked to look at the patient. The most commonly presented short case is Huntington's chorea, to see whether the candidate can recognize the abnormal movements associated with this disease. Rarely a younger patient with rheumatic chorea may be encountered as well.

- Look carefully for these abnormal quasipurposive rapid jerking movements affecting the face, tongue and the distal parts of the arms and legs. Rarely the movements may be limited to only one side of the body and then the condition is called hemichorea.
- Ask the patient to put the tongue out and notice that the patient will find it very difficult to keep it steady even for a short period.
- Ask the patient 'How are you?' and note the dysarthria with a slow and slurred speech.
- Ask for the permission of the examiner whether you could test the mental score of the patient by asking some simple questions. If low, this may be due to dementia which is a feature of Huntington's chorea.

Common questions

Q. What is the inheritance of Huntington's chorea?
A. Autosomal dominant.

Q. What are the other causes of chorea?
A. (i) Rheumatic chorea.
(ii) Chorea gravidarum.
(iii) Senile chorea.
(iv) Wilson's disease (cirrhosis, Kayser–Fleischer rings in cornea).

Q. Where is the lesion in chorea?
A. In basal ganglia.

23. Hemiballismus

You may be asked to look at the patient to check whether you recognize these involuntary movements.

- Note the violent, rapid flinging limb movement from full extension into abduction or external or internal rotation. Ballism is bilateral but hemiballism is confined to one side of the body. Once seen such movements are not usually forgotten.
- Sometimes there are similar abnormal movements of the head as well.

Common question

Q. Where is the lesion in such patients?
A. The lesion is thought to be in the subthalamic nucleus.

24. Titubation

You may be asked to look at a patient with these involuntary movements.

- Note the vertical oscillation of the head as the patient is sitting or standing. These movements disappear if the patient is lying down.
- Look for nystagmus and pallor of the optic discs.
- Look for intention tremor on finger–nose testing.
- Ask the patient to walk, and note the ataxic gait.
- Ask the patient, with the prior permission of the examiner, his address – and note the scanning character of his speech.

Common question

Q. Where is the lesion in patients with titubation?
A. Titubation indicates disease of the cerebellar connections, and is most commonly seen in multiple sclerosis.

25. Pigmentation of the mouth

You may be asked to look at a patient with Addison's disease.

- Note the brown or grey discoloration of the mucous surface of the lips and buccal mucosa, especially the inner aspect of the cheeks. Also, there may be pigmentation of the palate, gums and sides of the tongue.
- Note the hyperpigmentation of the exposed parts of the body, e.g. palmar creases, hands, arms, face and neck. Nipples and genitalia are also excessively pigmented.
- Note that the blood pressure is low, and check for postural hypotension.
- Note that the patient looks asthenic and, if a female, there may be loss of hair, both axillary and pubic.

Common questions

Q. What are the other causes of pigmentation of the mouth?
A. (i) Familial intestinal polyposis (Peutz–Jegher syndrome).
(ii) Racial.
(iii) Arsenic, bismuth or silver intake.
(iv) Metastatic malignant melanoma.

Q. Tell me something about Peutz–Jegher syndrome.
A. It is an autosomal dominant condition, characterized by the presence of mucocutaneous pigmentation of the lips, buccal mucosa, palms, toes and umbilical area, along with the presence of multiple polyps in the small intestine. Unlike familial polyposis coli, it is not a pre-malignant condition therefore, usually, no prophylactic excision of the polyps is advised.

Q. What is the cause of pigmentation in Addison's disease?
A. Pigmentation is caused both by excess of melanocyte stimulating hormone (MSH) and ACTH. The lower the cortisol secretion, the higher is the ACTH and MSH level.

Q. What single investigation should you want to do for Addison's disease?
A. Synacthen test.

26. Looking at the tongue

Occasionally you may be asked to comment upon the appearance of the tongue. Be familiar with the following conditions:

(a) Pallor of the tongue
This indicates anaemia and may be associated with atrophy of the filiform papillae resulting in a smooth, clean-looking tongue which may be caused by iron or vitamin B deficiency.

(b) Enlarged tongue
May be seen in cases of amyloidosis, acromegaly and myxoedema and if so look for the features of such conditions.

(c) Black hairy tongue
This is commonly due to fungal infection. The patient may be a heavy smoker on steroids or antibiotics in some cases. In candidiasis (thrush) creamy white patches appear on the tongue which can be easily scraped off.

(d) Geographical tongue
Disappearance of patches of papillae, leaving smooth areas on the tongue. This type of tongue has no clinical significance.

(e) Leukoplakia
This type of tongue is characterized by a painless, whitish patch which cannot be wiped off. This is a pre-cancerous condition.

(f) Some neurological conditions, like fasciculation of the tongue with wasting, may be seen in lower motor neurone disease such as progressive bulbar palsy, whereas spastic tongue with dysarthria and increased jaw jerk will be seen as a result of pseudobulbar palsy.

27. Neurofibromatosis

You may be asked to do a general physical examination or to examine a subcutaneous lump.

Locally

- Look for the cutaneous fibromas commonly seen on the trunk which are discrete, moveable lumps arranged along lines of nerves. Sometimes they may be painful or tender on pressure.
- Look for the café-au-lait spots, which are coloured patches of skin pigmentation. Pigmentation is most prominent over the trunk. Axillary freckling is commonly seen.
- Look for kyphoscoliosis.

Elsewhere

- Look for deafness and cerebellar signs (ataxia, nystagmus and scanning speech) for acoustic neuroma which may be seen in a patient with neurofibromatosis.
- Mention the need for checking blood pressure as phaeochromocytoma (causing hypertension) is rarely associated with neurofibromatosis.

Common question

Q. What is the treatment of this condition?
A. No treatment is required unless a localized tumour causes cerebral or spinal compression. If the patient is hypertensive, phaeochromocytoma should be strongly suspected. Phaeochromocytomas, intracranial and spinal tumours require surgery.

28. Lymphadenopathy

You may be asked to examine the lymphatic system of a particular patient.

- Do not forget to examine pre- and post-auricular, submental, tonsillar and occipital lymph nodes, along with detection of enlarged supraclavicular lymph nodes in the head and neck area.
- In the upper limb always look for enlargement of epitrochlear lymph nodes.

- Now examine both axillae and groins for any lymphadeno-pathy.
- Do not forget to examine the abdomen for any enlargement of paraaortic or iliac lymph nodes and hepatic or splenomegaly.
- Always look for consistency, tenderness and matting of the lymph nodes which helps in deciding about the possible cause of lymphadenopathy.

Common question

Q. What are the causes for generalized lymphadenopathy?
A. (i) Acute and chronic leukaemias.
   (ii) Lymphoma.
   (iii) Infections, e.g. infectious mononucleosis, secondary syphilis and miliary tuberculosis.
   (iv) Collagen diseases, e.g. systemic lupus erythematosus, Still's disease and rheumatoid arthritis.
   (v) Other conditions, e.g. sarcoidosis.

29. Superior vena cava syndrome

A patient with such a syndrome who has recently been started on radiotherapy treatment may be shown as a short case.

- Note the conjunctival suffusion and brawny oedema of the face, neck, upper arms and thorax.
- Note the prominent veins over the upper trunk with blood flowing downwards (due to the development of numerous superficial collateral vessels).
- Note the prominent and distended jugular veins.
- Note any marking of the area of radiotherapy.
- Test for hoarseness as another sign for metastatic manifestation.
- Look for finger clubbing of the nails.
- Examine the chest for signs of carcinoma of the lung, e.g. collapse, consolidation, pleural effusion, etc.

Common question

Q. How does carcinoma of the lung cause this syndrome?

A. Metastases in mediastinal lymph nodes cause compression or invasion of the superior vena cava and thus interferes with the venous return.

30. Goitre

Any enlargement of the thyroid gland is described as goitre and you may be asked to look at the neck.

• Note the swelling of the thyroid gland and check whether the swelling moves on deglutition.

• Palpate both from the front and behind the patient to determine the size, shape, consistency and extent of the swelling, including any possible retrosternal extension.

• Check for any signs of compression of the trachea, recurrent laryngeal nerve (ask for any difficulty in swallowing and speech) and superior vena cava (see Case 29).

• Listen carefully for any bruit over the gland. If present this suggests hyperactivity of the gland.

• Look for any enlarged lymph nodes in the neck which may mean metastasis from carcinoma of the thyroid.

• Look for other signs of thyrotoxicosis (staring look of the patient with exophthalmos, lid-lag, tremors and pretibial myxoedema), or of hypothyroidism (coarse features with dry skin, slow pulse and slow relaxation of ankle jerk).

Discussion and common questions

Please see Cases 4 and 5.

31. Gynaecomastia

You may be asked to examine the chest of a male patient. The only finding may be enlargement of the breasts. In any case make sure that this is definite breast tissue and not simply excessive fat deposition in an obese person.

- If the person is very tall, look for features of Kleinfelter's syndrome (see Case 8).
- Look for stigmata of cirrhosis of liver since gynaecomastia may be one of the features of cirrhosis.
- Palpate and look for any testicular tumour, as rarely this can cause gynaecomastia.
- Look for rare conditions which may account for gynaecomastia, e.g. acromegaly, thyrotoxicosis and Addison's disease.

Common question

Q. What drugs can cause gynaecomastia?
A. (i) Digitalis.
   (ii) Spironolactone.
   (iii) Oestrogens.
   (iv) Steroids.
   (v) Phenothiazines.
   (vi) Cimetidine.
   (vii) Methyldopa.
   (viii) Reserpine.

Cardiovascular System

32. Mitral stenosis

Locally

- Note that the apex beat is tapping in character with a para-sternal heave, due to right ventricular enlargement. Also feel for a diastolic thrill at the apex.
- The murmur is an apical rough rumbling mid-diastolic one and best heard in the left lateral recumbent position. If the patient is in sinus rhythm, there may be presystolic accentuation of the murmur. Exercising the patient makes the murmur more prominent. With the onset of fibrillation, the presystolic accentuation disappears.
- Note that the first heart sound is loud and just after the second sound there is a localized, sharp, short, high-pitched sound, called the opening snap. It is best heard at or just inside the apex beat. With severe stenosis, the opening snap follows closely on the second sound, but with mild stenosis it is delayed.
- Check if there is more than one valvular lesion and if mitral incompetence is also present, decide which one is the dominant lesion. Loud first heart sound with the presence of opening snap favour mitral stenosis, whereas a faint first heart sound accompanied with third heart sound is more suggestive of mitral incompetence.

Elsewhere

- Look for malar flush. Remember malar flush is also present with other conditions causing pulmonary hypertension.
- Examine the pulse which is usually normal volume, but rarely with severe degree of stenosis may be of small volume.
- Look for any signs of congestive cardiac failure and JVP 'a' waves indicating pulmonary hypertension.
- Look for signs of infective endocarditis, e.g. clubbing, petechial haemorrhages, splinter nails, clubbing and splenomegaly, etc.

Discussion

The murmur of mitral stenosis is best heard by asking the patient to exercise and then turning on to his left side. The pulse may or may not be of small volume, but will never be of large volume in pure mitral stenosis.

Common questions

Q. How do you decide about the severity of the stenosis?
A. (i) The longer the diastolic murmur, the severer is the stenosis. The duration and not the intensity of the murmur matters. If the patient is in sinus rhythm there is a presystolic accentuation of the mid-diastolic murmur.
(ii) The shorter the interval between the second heart sound and the opening snap, the more marked the stenosis.
(iii) Jugular venous pressure 'a' waves, loud P_2, right ventricular hypertrophy with P pulmonale on ECG, and Kerley's B lines with or without pulmonary oedema on CXR: all favour a severe mitral stenosis.

Q. How is the patient affected on developing atrial fibrillation?
A. (i) Chances of heart failure are increased.
(ii) Chances of infective endocarditis are decreased.
(iii) Presystolic accentuation disappears.
(iv) Thromboembolism with stroke, etc.

33. Mitral incompetence

Locally

- Note that the apex beat is displaced to the left and downwards and is strong and localized, suggesting left ventricular hypertrophy.
- Feel for the presence of a systolic thrill at the apex.
- On auscultation confirm whether the patient is in sinus rhythm or not. You would expect to hear a pansystolic atrial murmur radiating to the left axilla. The first heart sound is unusually quiet, but often a 3rd beat sound is present due to the increased return of the regurgitated blood from the left atrium.
- Search for any evidence of pulmonary hypertension, e.g. parasternal heave and a loud P_2.
- Look for any other associated valvular disease – most commonly mitral stenosis in cases of rheumatic heart disease.

Elsewhere

- In all cardiovascular conditions the peripheral signs must be looked for first before you actually start examining the heart itself (unless the examiner indicates otherwise).
- Pulse – its volume, regularity and the character. With slow atrial fibrillation the irregularities of the pulse become difficult to detect.
- Hands – Marfan's syndrome – arachnodactyly.
- Malar flush.

Discussion

In uncomplicated mitral incompetence the apical first sound is faint, and is replaced by a loud blowing, pansystolic murmur extending into the axilla. The apex beat is strong and localized, suggesting left ventricular hypertrophy. Chest X-ray shows enlarged left ventricle and atrium. Early symptoms are easy fatiguability and exertional and nocturnal dyspnoea.

Common questions

Q. What are the four important causes of mitral incompetence?

A. (i) Rheumatic heart disease.

(ii) Papillary muscle dysfunction due to coronary heart disease.

(iii) Left ventricular hypertrophy with dilatation of mitral ring.

(iv) Prolapsed mitral valve (congenital).

Q. Why is this murmur not a murmur of VSD or tricuspid incompetence?

A. VSD murmur does not radiate to the left axilla. Tricuspid incompetence is accompanied by a giant V wave in the JVP and systolic pulsation of an enlarged liver. Moreover, the murmur of tricuspid incompetence increases during inspiration due to increased ventricular filling, whereas the pansystolic murmur of mitral incompetence increases during expiration.

Q. Do you think that mitral incompetence is haemodynamically significant?

A. Yes, if the incompetence is accompanied by left ventricular enlargement.

34. Aortic stenosis

Locally

• Ejection mid-systolic murmur heard loudest at the base, usually, but not necessarily, conducted to the right side of the neck. It may be heard over the whole of the precordium. The second aortic sound is absent or diminished.

• Heaving displaced apex beat suggestive of left ventricular hypertrophy. Also, a systolic thrill may be present.

• Any other associated valvular lesion.

Elsewhere

- Like other cardiovascular cases, peripheral signs are very important and one is well advised to start by examining the pulse – volume, regularity and character. The pulse is of small amplitude and rises slowly to a delayed peak with a slow fall. There may be an extra impulse felt at the peak and then it is called anacrotic pulse, which is considered to be diagnostic of aortic stenosis.
- Look for signs of left ventricular failure.

Discussion

As in all cases, the candidate must go over the ritual of inspection (apex beat), palpation (apex beat/thrills) and auscultation. Percussion is not thought to be very helpful and may even be omitted. Aortic sclerosis, due to atherosclerotic hardening of the cusps of the aortic valve without gross narrowing, is a common condition and should be differentiated from true aortic stenosis. The pulse remains of normal volume and character in aortic sclerosis, whereas is anacrotic in aortic stenosis.

Common questions

Q. How can the patient present?
A. (i) Angina.
(ii) Syncopal attacks.
(iii) Clinical features of left ventricular failure.

Q. What are the common causes of aortic stenosis?
A. (i) Rheumatic heart disease.
(ii) Congenital (especially in the younger patient without any other valvular lesion).
(iii) In elderly males it is usually due to calcification of congenital bicuspid aortic valve.

35. Aortic incompetence

Locally

- The cardinal sign is the presence of an early diastolic murmur, best heard at the left sternal edge (right sternal edge in Marfan's syndrome and syphilitic aortitis) with the patient sitting up and holding his breath at the height of expiration.
- Signs of other associated valvular lesions.

Elsewhere

- As in all other cardiovascular cases, always start with the pulse – volume, regularity and character, e.g. collapsing (water hammer) pulse. But do remember that the absence of collapsing pulse does not rule out aortic incompetence. A pulse with double peak is called pulsus bisferiens, and is due to combined aortic stenosis and incompetence.
- Collapsing pulsation in the neck arising from the carotid arteries (Corrigan's sign).
- Look for other stigmata of syphilis, such as Argyll Robertson pupil and ptosis.
- Signs of left ventricular failure.

Discussion

Many patients with aortic incompetence are asymptomatic for decades. With progressive regurgitation, left ventricular dilation and eventually left ventricular failure ensues. Some other signs of aortic incompetence such as pistol shots (sounds auscultated over femoral artery) and Duroziez murmurs (to and fro murmur audible on slight compression of femoral artery) are less important and do not really contribute much to the diagnosis. The candidate, therefore, must not waste time on such less significant signs.

Common questions

Q. What are the causes of aortic incompetence?
A. (i) Rheumatic heart disease.
   (ii) Syphilis.

34

(iii) Ankylosing spondylitis.

(iv) Marfan's syndrome.

(v) Infective endocarditis.

Q. What are other causes for water hammer pulse?

A. (i) Anaemia.

(ii) Thyrotoxicosis.

(iii) Paget's disease of the bone.

(iv) High fever.

(v) Pregnancy.

36. Coarctation of aorta

You may be asked to examine the cardiovascular system.

Locally (*Nb.* like other cardiovascular cases always start with the examination of the pulse.)

• Systolic murmur over the precordium with or without cardiac enlargement.

• Look for visible/palpable arterial pulsation on the back which is best seen with the patient leaning forward.

Elsewhere

• Palpate both radial and femoral pulsations simultaneously.

• The femoral pulsations are markedly diminished and delayed in coarctation of aorta when compared with the radial pulses.

• Confirm by taking blood pressure (with the permission of the examiner) both in upper and lower limbs: the readings will be much lower in the lower limbs.

Discussion

The diagnosis of this tricky short case can be easily missed unless the candidate keeps a strict practice of palpating the femoral pulsations along with radial arteries on both sides. Coarctation is much more common in men, and in women with Turner's syndrome. The possibility of coarctation should always be considered in any hypertensive patient under the age of forty-five. The usual causes of death in untreated cases are bacterial endocarditis and ruptured cerebral aneurysm.

Common questions

Q. What single most important investigation would you ask for?
A. CXR. (Look for rib notching.)

Q. What are the other causes of rib notching?
A. (i) Neurofibromatosis.
   (ii) Inferior vena cava obstruction.

Q. What are the four signs commonly seen in the CXR?
A. (i) Notching of the ribs.
   (ii) Dilated ascending aorta.
   (iii) Figures of '3' sign due to indentation of the aorta at the site of coarctation with pre- and poststenotic dilatation.
   (iv) Dilated left subclavian artery.

37. Atrial septal defect

Locally

- The apex beat is not usually displaced but in some cases there may be a left parasternal heave due to the right ventricular enlargement.
- Listen carefully for a mid-systolic murmur left of the sternum maximal in the 3rd intercostal space with wide splitting of the second heart sound which is relatively fixed in relation to respiration.
- Rarely mitral stenosis may be associated with ASD so listen for a mid-diastolic murmur of the mitral stenosis, if present (Lutembacher's syndrome).

Elsewhere

- Examine the radial pulse as usual (usually large volume pulse).

- Look for dyspnoea, cyanosis, raised JVP, liver enlargement and oedema of the feet, signs of heart failure in cases of ASD with reversed shunts.
- Look for any signs of infective endocarditis (rare in cases of ASD) e.g. clubbing of the nails, splinter haemorrhages, anaemia and splenomegaly, etc.

Common question

Q. What three investigations would you like to ask for?
A. (i) ECG: incomplete right bundle branch block is quite common in ostium secundum defects, whereas in primum defect it may be left bundle branch block.
(ii) CXR: cardiomegaly with pulmonary plethora (hilar dance).
(iii) Cardiac catheterization.

38. Ventricular septal defect

You may be asked to listen to the heart or examine the cardio-vascular system.

Locally

- The apex beat is usually not displaced.
- Palpate for a systolic thrill maximal in the 4th intercostal space to the left of the sternum.
- On auscultation you would expect to hear a pansystolic murmur best heard in the 3rd or 4th left intercostal space radiating over the precordium.
- Also listen carefully for the presence of a third heart sound which is often present and is due to rapid filling of the left ventricle.
- Listen for the presence of any functional pulmonary systolic or mitral diastolic murmurs which may be seen in patients with larger septal defects where the output of the right ventricle may be even double that of the left ventricle into the aorta.

Elsewhere

- Examine the radial pulse as for other cardiovascular cases.
- Look for central cyanosis which is seen in cases of VSD with reversed shunts (Eisenmenger's syndrome).
- Look for any evidence of congestive cardiac failure e.g. raised JVP, liver enlargement or oedema of the feet.
- Look for any evidence of infective endocarditis e.g. clubbing, splinter haemorrhages, anaemia, pyrexia and splenomegaly etc.

Common questions

Q. What is Maladie de Roger?

A. When VSD is so small that it is asymptomatic, and not accompanied by any change in the ECG or chest X-ray, it is called Maladie de Roger. A small VSD gives a loud murmur and with larger shunts the murmur may become less pronounced.

Q. What are the indication and contraindication for surgery of VSD?

A. *Indications:*
   (i) If right ventricular systolic pressure exceeds 50 mm of Hg.
   (ii) Pulmonary to systemic flow ratio in excess of 1.5 to 1.7.
   Contra-indication:
   Eisenmenger's syndrome.

Respiratory System

39. Collapse of the lung

You may be asked to examine the chest of a patient with collapse of a lobe of the lung.

Locally

Inspection
- Diminished chest movement with flattening of the chest wall on the side of the collapse.

Palpation
- Trachea and the apex beat of the heart of shifted towards the side of the lesion.

Percussion
- Percussion note is impaired.

Auscultation
- Impaired breath sounds.
- Bronchial breathing and crepitations may be present if associated with consolidation.

Discussion

The shift of the trachea is seen if the upper lobe of the lung is collapsed, whereas if the lower lobe is collapsed it is the apex beat that is shifted towards the side of the collapse. In the chest X-ray, the area of collapse of the lung is seen as a homogeneous dense opacity. A lateral film may help to locate the lobes affected by collapse.

Common questions

Q. What are the causes of collapse of the lung?
A. (i) Obstruction of a major bronchus by malignancy, foreign body, enlarged lymph node or pus.
(ii) Compression of the lung by pleural effusion or pneumo-thorax.

Q. What three investigations do you want to do?
A. (i) Chest X-ray.
(ii) Sputum for AFB, malignant cells, culture and sensitivity.
(iii) Bronchoscopy.

40. Consolidation of the lung

Locally

Inspection
- Note that the movement of the chest wall is reduced on the affected side.
- No shift of trachea or apex beat.

Palpation
- Vocal fremitus is increased.
- Look for lymphadenopathy in the axillae and the neck.

Percussion
- Percussion note is impaired.

Auscultation
- Bronchial breathing.
- Fine or coarse crepitations.
- Pleural rub may be present.
- Vocal resonance is increased.
- Listen carefully for the presence of whispering pectoriloquy.

Elsewhere

- Look for cyanosis.
- Examine pulse. Usually tachycardia.
- Look for clubbing of the fingers.

Discussion

Consolidation simply means an area of pneumonia. On a chest X-ray there is a homogeneous opacity with ill-defined margins. A lateral film usually helps to locate the lobes affected by consolidation. In pure consolidation a tracheal or mediastinal shift is not expected. Clubbing of the fingers may be seen if the consolidation is due to bronchial carcinoma.

Common questions

Q. What are the causes of consolidation?
A. (i) Infection.
   (ii) Infarction.
   (iii) Malignancy.

Q. What three investigations do you want to do?
A. (i) Chest X-ray.
   (ii) Sputum for AFB, malignant cells, culture and sensivity.
   (iii) Bronchoscopy.

41. Pleural effusion

Locally

Inspection
- Diminished chest movement on the side of the effusion.

Palpation
- Trachea and the apex beat of the heart are not shifted until the effusion is massive.
- Vocal fremitus is impaired or absent.

Percussion
- Stony dullness over the effusion.

Auscultation
- Absent or reduced intensity of breathing.
- Vocal resonance is usually absent.
- Bronchial breathing may be present over the upper limit of the effusion.

Elsewhere

- Look for possible causes of effusion, e.g. rheumatoid arthritis (joints), systemic lupus erythematosus (butterfly rash).

Discussion

With the patient sitting up, the rising dullness of the pleural fluid can be demonstrated in patients with pleural effusion. In the chest X-ray, the opacity seems to rise laterally. On lateral view it shows that the opacity is not segmental or lobar in distribution, but is usually unnecessary.

Common questions

Q. What are the common causes of pleural effusion?
A. (i) Heart failure.
(ii) Infection, e.g. pneumonia, TB.
(iii) Infarction.
(iv) Malignancy.

Q. What investigations would you ask for?
A. (i) Chest X-ray.
(ii) Aspiration of pleural fluid for cytology, AFB and biochemistry for protein content.
(iii) Sputum for AFB, malignant cells, culture and sensitivity.
(iv) Pleural biopsy.

Q. What is the difference between a transudate and an exudate?
A. The transudate has low protein content (less than 20 g l⁻¹) and is usually seen with heart failure, renal and liver disease and Meig's syndrome. The exudate has a high protein content (more than 20 g l⁻¹) and is usually seen in cases of infection, infarction and malignancy of lung.

42. Fibrosing alveolitis

You may be asked to listen to the back of the chest, for example, where you may find fine basal crepitations usually on both sides.

• Look for other features, e.g. dyspnoea, clubbing and cyanosis.
• Look for features of right sided heart failure (cor pulmonale), e.g. raised JVP, hepatomegaly and pitting oedema in the legs.

Discussion

Idiopathic diffuse interstitial fibrosis or fibrosing alveolitis is a condition characterized by dyspnoea, dry cough, clubbing of fingers and crepitations mainly over lower portions of lungs. Some patients with rheumatoid arthritis develop similar fibrosis over the base of the lungs, but in ankylosing spondylitis the fibrosis is seen in only the upper portions of the lungs. Other collagen disorders causing interstitial pulmonary fibrosis include scleroderma and dermatomyositis.

Common question

Q. What investigations would you ask for?
A. (i) Lung function tests including transfer factor.
(ii) Serum autoantibodies – antinuclear factors and rheumatoid factor.
(iii) Blood gases.
(iv) Needle biopsy of the lung.

43. Kyphoscoliosis

Rarely you may be asked to examine the chest of a patient where the only abnormality may be kyphoscoliosis.

• Note whether the kyphoscoliosis is mainly in the thoracic region or thoracolumbar region.
• Look for any hump or gibbus formation due to the rotation of the spine with prominence of the posterior angles of the ribs.
• Note and describe whether the curvature of the scoliosis is to

the left or to the right, besides looking for fused vertebrae, spina bifida and absent ribs.

- Look for other features of certain conditions commonly associated with kyphoscoliosis, e.g. Marfan's syndrome, neurofibromatosis.

- Look for any evidence of cardiopulmonary disability which may be caused or result from gross kyphoscoliosis.

Common question

Q. What two investigations would you ask for?
A. (i) Chest X-ray.
   (ii) Lung function tests.

Abdomen

44. Hepatomegaly

Locally

- Describe the extent of enlargement, preferably in centimetres or inches, and not in finger breadth.
- Edge of liver – regular or irregular.
- Surface – smooth or nodular.
- Consistency – firm or hard.
- Tenderness – present or not.
- Always percuss both the lower and upper borders (normally dull up to 4th intercostal space).
- Auscultate for any bruits or rub.
- Check for any splenomegaly.
- Check for ascites and caput medusae.

Elsewhere

- Look for lymphadenopathy.
- Spider naevi.
- Leuconychia.
- Raised JVP.
- Jaundice.
- Gynaecomastia.
- Testicular atrophy.
- Oedema of feet.
- Absence of secondary sexual hair.

45

Common conditions

- Congestive cardiac failure.
- Cirrhosis (alcoholic).
- Carcinoma of liver (secondaries most commonly).
- Lymphoma.
- Infective hepatitis.

Discussion

In such a short case it is important to know not only the extent of liver enlargement but to look for important associated features of certain conditions mentioned above. Relevant features for congestive cardiac failure would be a raised jugular venous pressure and oedema of the feet, along with an enlarged, firm, tender liver with a smooth surface and regular sharp edge. If the liver enlargement is due to cirrhosis, the consistency of the liver is hard and splenomegaly, ascites, spider naevi, Dupuytren's contracture and palmar erythema are commonly seen. A hard knobbly liver, with or without tenderness, is suggestive of carcinomatosis as the most probably cause of hepatomegaly.

Common question

Q. What investigations would you ask for?
A. (i) Liver function tests.
   (ii) Liver scan.
   (iii) Australian antigen.
   (iv) Alphafetoprotein.
   (v) Liver biopsy.

45. Splenomegaly

Locally

- Describe how much enlarged (centimetres or inches).
- Look for hepatomegaly.
- Look for ascites.

Elsewhere

- Look for lymphadenopathy.
- Anaemia.
- Jaundice.
- Plethoric facies.
- Sternal tenderness.
- Splinter haemorrhages.
- Rheumatoid hands.

Common conditions

- (a) Mild enlargement of the spleen
  Viral hepatitis.
  Infectious mononucleosis.
  Septicaemia.
  Typhoid fever.
  Brucellosis.
  Systemic lupus erythematosus.
  Felty's syndrome.
- (b) Moderate enlargement of the spleen
  Chronic lymphatic leukaemia.
  Malignant lymphoma.
  Acute leukaemia.
  Anaemia
  (i) Aplastic.
  (ii) Pernicious.
  (iii) Haemolytic.
  Idiopathic thrombocytopaenic purpura.
  Biliary cirrhosis.
  Infective endocarditis.
  Sarcoidosis.
  Amyloidosis.
- (c) Massive enlargement of the spleen
  Chronic myeloid leukaemia.
  Myelofibrosis.
  Polycythaemia rubra vera.
  Malaria.
  Kala-azar.

Discussion

The candidate must always ask the patient to turn on to his right, so that the splenic notch can be easily palpable in cases where there is only a marginal enlargement of the spleen. For a mildly enlarged spleen lymphoma, anaemia and polycythaemia are important causes, and the presence or absence of coexisting features such as pallor, plethoric facies, liver enlargement or lymphadenopathy should help in deciding the most probable cause. Moderate to grossly enlarged spleens are commonly a result of myelofibrosis, chronic myeloid leukaemia or, rarely, due to malaria. Cirrhosis is the most likely cause of splenomegaly if associated with portal hypertension.

Common question

Q. What are the features of an enlarged spleen?
A. (i) Palpable splenic notch.
   (ii) Inability to get in below the costal margin.
   (iii) Not bimanually palpable, unlike enlarged kidney.
   (iv) Presence of dullness, unlike a band of resonance, over the kidney.
   (v) An enlarged spleen moves with respiration.
   (vi) The direction of the enlargement is medially.

46. Hepatosplenomegaly

Locally

- As described for hepatomegaly and splenomegaly determine their extent of enlargement.
- Look for ascites.

Elsewhere

- Lymphadenopathy.
- Spider naevi.
- Leuconychia.
- Raised JVP.

- Jaundice, anaemia.
- Sternal tenderness.
- Gynaecomastia.
- Testicular atrophy.
- Oedema of feet.

Common conditions

- Lymphoma.
- Leukaemia.
- Cirrhosis.
- Myeloproliferative disorders.

Discussion

The extent of the enlargement of the spleen and the liver usually are helpful in giving some clue to the cause of hepatosplenomegaly. In myelofibrosis and chronic myeloid leukaemia the spleen is markedly enlarged, whereas in acute leukaemia the enlargement is less than moderate. Cirrhosis, with all its stigmata of liver cell disease, remains a common short case.

Common questions

Q. What are the causes of portal hypertension?
A. (i) Cirrhosis of the liver.
   (ii) Hepatic vein obstruction (Budd Chiari syndrome).
   (iii) Constrictive pericarditis.

Q. What are the causes of ascites?
A. (i) *Transudation*
   Cirrhosis.
   Nephrotic syndrome.
   Congestive cardiac failure.
   (ii) *Exudation*
   Tubercular peritonitis.
   Carcinomatous peritonitis.
   (iii) *Chylous ascites*
   Malignancy.
   Trauma.

47. Renal enlargement

Locally

- Make sure that this is renal enlargement and not, for example, splenomegaly.
- See if the other kidney is enlarged as well.

Elsewhere

- Look for anaemia.
- Any puffiness around the eyelids?
- Does the patient look uraemic?
- Look for oedema of the legs.

Common conditions

- Polycystic disease of the kidney.
- Hydronephrosis.
- Renal tumour.
- Nephrotic syndrome.

Common questions

Q. How do you differentiate the kidney enlargement from splenomegaly?

A. *Kidney*	*Spleen*
Rounded border	Sharp edge
Possible to pass fingers between upper end of kidney and ribs	Not so
Bimanually palpable	Not so
Presence of colonic resonance anteriorly	Not so
Moves only slightly with respiration	Moves freely with respiration

Q. What four investigations would you ask for?
A. (i) Urine examination for protein, cells and casts, etc.
   (ii) IVP.
   (iii) Renal ultrasound.
   (iv) Renal angiography.

48. Ascites

You may be asked to examine the abdomen.

Locally

- Note carefully the distension of the abdomen with fullness in the flanks.
- Look for any dilated veins over the abdomen and if present determine the direction of flow of blood in these veins.
- Look for any liver or splenic enlargement. Sometimes with gross ascites this may be very difficult. 'Dipping' over these organs may be helpful.
- Look for the presence of fluid thrill.
- Look for shifting dullness to confirm the ascites.

Elsewhere

- Look for stigmata of cirrhosis, e.g. Dupuytren's contracture, palmar erythema, spider naevi, etc.
- Look for signs of congestive cardiac failure and constrictive pericarditis, e.g. raised JVP and oedema of the legs.
- Intra-abdominal causes include carcinomatosis or tuberculosis of the peritoneum and the nephrotic syndrome.

Common question

Q. What two investigations would you like to do?
A. (i) Ascitic fluid for protein content, cytology, culture and acid fast bacilli.
   (ii) Abdominal ultrasound.

49. Mass in the epigastrium

You may be asked to feel the tummy.

Locally

Inspection
- See if there is any visible distension in the epigastric region.
- Look for any visible peristalsis.
- Movement with respiration?

Palpation
- Define the consistency and the size of the mass.
- Make sure this is not an enlarged left lobe of the liver or enlarged spleen.

Percussion
- Check for gastric splash.
- Check for expansibility or transmitted pulsations.
- Look for fluid thrill which may be present in large pancreatic cysts.

Auscultation
- Listen to the bowel sounds.
- Any bruit over the mass?

Elsewhere

- Is the patient cachectic?
- Jaundice (pancreatic tumour)?
- Anaemia?
- Left supraclavicular gland enlargement (carcinoma of the stomach)?

Common conditions

- Carcinoma of the stomach.
- Carcinoma of the transverse colon.
- Aneurysm of abdominal aorta.
- Pancreatic tumour or pseudocyst.

• Retroperitoneal lymphadenopathy.

Common question

Q. What investigations you would ask for?
A. (i) Barium-meal.
   (ii) Abdominal ultrasound.
   (iii) CT scan of abdomen.
   (iv) Endoscopy.

50. Mass in right iliac fossa

Locally

Inspection
• Look for any visible swelling.
• Any visible peristalsis?
• Presence of sinuses over the skin (actinomycosis, TB or Crohn's disease)?

Palpation
• Define size, surface, consistency and tenderness of the mass.

Auscultation
• Bowel sounds.

Elsewhere

• Anaemia.
• Lymphadenopathy.
• Clubbing (Crohn's disease).

Common conditions

• Crohn's disease.
• Appendicular mass.
• Tubo-ovarian mass.
• Carcinoid tumour.
• TB, amoeboma rarely.

Common question

Q. What investigations would you ask for?
A. (i) Abdominal ultrasound.
   (ii) Barium-meal follow through (Crohn's disease/TB).
   (iii) Ultrasound for ovarian mass.
   (iv) 5 HIAA (raised in carcinoid syndrome).
   (v) Stools for amoebae (amoeboma).

51. Dilated abdominal wall veins

Locally

• Note the dilated and prominent veins around the umbilicus.
• Demonstrate the direction of blood flow.
• Look for hepatosplenomegaly.
• Look for ascites.

Elsewhere

• Spider naevi.
• Palmar erythema.
• Dupuytren's contracture.
• Leuconychia.
• Oedema of legs (hypoproteinaemia).
• Absence of secondary sexual hair.

Common conditions

• Cirrhosis of liver.
• Inferior vena caval obstruction.

Discussion

Distended veins radiating from the umbilicus are called caput medusae. Portal obstruction resulting in the establishment of a connection between the portal and parietal veins by means of round ligament is the explanation for these dilated veins. You must learn and practise demonstrating the direction of blood flow in these veins. Above the umbilicus it is upwards towards the thorax, and below the umbilicus it is downwards towards the groin, i.e. away from the umbilicus in all directions. In inferior vena caval obstruction, the collateral veins carry blood upwards to reach the superior vena caval system.

Common question

Q. What are the causes of inferior vena caval obstruction?

A. (i) Tumour obstructing the blood flow.

(ii) Trauma.

(iii) Thrombosis.

Central Nervous System

52. Pseudobulbar palsy

You may be asked to look at the patient or to examine the cranial nerves.

- Note the emotional lability of the patient. The patient may have a peculiar facial expression and laugh or cry for no apparent reasons.
- Ask the patient to protrude the tongue and note that this can only be achieved with difficulty, because of the spasticity and the stiffness of the tongue.
- Test for the movement of the soft palate and note that the palate is paralysed.
- Demonstrate the briskness of the jaw jerk.
- Ask the patient about his address and notice the dysarthria.
- Look for the presence of fasciculations in the limb muscles (motor neurone disease).
- Look for upper motor neurone signs in the limbs usually more marked in lower limbs with spasticity, brisk reflexes and up-going plantars.

Common questions

Q. What are the causes of pseudobulbar palsy?
A. (i) Bilateral cerebrovascular accidents.   *MS .*
   (ii) Motor neurone disease. *V. uncommon.*

MND man LMN lesion. More likely to get bulbar palsy

56

(iii) Multiple sclerosis.

Q. What is bulbar palsy?

A. This condition is less common than pseudobulbar palsy, characterized by bilateral wasting of the tongue with fasciculation, paralysis of the palate, dysarthria and, rarely, extraocular muscle palsy. This is due to lower motor neurone type of lesion and may be caused by motor neurone disease or syringobulbia.

53. 3rd Nerve palsy

Locally

Note that the eyeball is rotated outwards (by the unopposed action of lateral rectus) and downwards (by the unopposed action of superior oblique).

- Note the ptosis which is due to drooping of the levator palpabris superioris.
- Note that the pupil is dilated (due to unopposed action of the sympathetic impulses) with loss of light and accommodation reflex.
- Test the functions of the muscles supplied by the 3rd nerve, and you will find that the eyeball fails to move in other directions.

Common questions

Q. What is ptosis?

A. Drooping of the eyelid is called ptosis. Normally only the upper one-sixth of the cornea is covered by the eyelid; more than that is ptosis.

Q. What are the important causes of 3rd nerve palsy?

A. (i) Vascular lesion e.g. thrombosis, aneurysm and haemorrhage.
(ii) Neoplasm.
(iii) Diabetes mellitus.
(iv) Multiple sclerosis.

Q. Tell me about the lesions affecting the 3rd nerve during its course.

A. Since the two nuclei lie close together, a nuclear lesion may affect both the 3rd nerves and the ptosis is partial in these lesions. Multiple sclerosis, neoplasm and haemorrhage commonly affect the 3rd nerve at its origin. If the lesion is in the base of the midbrain it commonly causes 3rd nerve palsy with crossed hemiplegia due to involvement of costicospinal tracts (Weber's syndrome). In the interpeduncular space, aneurysm at the junction of the posterior cerebral artery with the posterior communicating artery may compress the 3rd nerve. Further in its course, cavernous sinus lesions involve the 4th nerve and ophthalmic division of the 5th and 6th nerves, along with the 3rd nerve. Similarly, within the orbit, fractures or retro-orbital swellings also involve ophthalmic division of the 5th and 6th cranial nerves along with the 3rd nerve.

54. 6th Nerve palsy

You may be asked to look at the patient or to examine the eyes.

• Note the deviation of the eyeball medially (convergent squint) of the affected eye. This is due to the unopposed action of the medial rectus muscle.

• Now test the various movements of each eye separately by asking the patient to follow your finger in all directions. In cases of 6th nerve palsy, the eyeball on the affected side fails to move laterally, due to the paralysis of the external rectus. Also, the patient will experience diplopia when trying to move the eye in the direction of the paralysed muscle.

Common question

Q. What are the common causes of 6th nerve palsy?
A. (i) Raised intracranial pressure (due to the stretching of the nerve) and, thus, a false localizing sign.

(ii) Vascular lesion, e.g. aneurysm of the internal carotid artery.
(iii) Neoplasm.
(iv) Encephalitis.
(v) Multiple sclerosis.

55. Facial (7th) nerve palsy

You may be asked to look at the face.

- Note the loss of nasolabial fold and the asymmetrical face on either side.
- Ascertain whether this involves the lower half of the face (UMN lesion), or a complete half of the face (LMN lesion). This can be done by asking the patient to produce furrows over the forehead, blowing out the cheeks, closing the eyes tightly, whistling and smiling.

UMN type of facial palsy

- Look carefully for the presence of associated hemiparesis, as a patient with UMN facial palsy would very commonly have a stroke on the same side, with or without speech difficulties.

LMN type of facial involvement

- Look for any parotid swelling (tumour).
- Look behind the ear for any scar of operation on the mastoid.
- Look for any evidence of sarcoidosis on the face such as lupus pernio plaques etc. Remember sarcoidosis may cause bilateral facial LMN type of palsy.

Common question

Q. What are the other causes of facial (LMN type) palsy.
A. (i) Bell's palsy.
   (ii) Multiple sclerosis.
   (iii) Neoplasm (acoustic neuroma).

56. Exophthalmos or proptosis

You may be asked to look at the patient.

Locally

Note the undue prominence of the eyeballs. If in doubt examine the patient in profile and from above:

- Note the lid retraction with wide palpebral fissure.
- Test for the presence of lid-lag.
- Check the movements of the eyeballs to rule out exophthalmic ophthalmoplegia.
- Listen for any bruit over the eyeball.

Elsewhere

- In the neck, look for any thyroid enlargement.
- Ask the patient to spread the fingers and look for the presence of fine tremors.
- Look for pretibial myxoedema.
- Examine the cardiovascular system for presence of tachycardia, atrial fibrillation.

Common questions

Q. What are the causes of unilateral exophthalmos?
A. (i) Thyrotoxicosis (early stage).
(ii) Retro-orbital tumours or cellulitis.
(iii) Cavernous sinus thrombosis – usually seen with marked chemosis and ophthalmoplegia.

Q. How is progressive exophthalmos treated?
A. *Medical measures*
(i) Sunglasses to protect eyes from dust and foreign bodies.
(ii) Methyl cellulose 1% eye drops to prevent corneal dryness.
(iii) Diuretics to reduce orbital oedema.
(iv) Steroids in high doses.
Surgical measures
(i) Tarsorrhaphy.
(ii) Orbital decompression.

57. Squint

Squint or strabismus is a deviation of the eye from the optical axis. When you are dealing with a case of squint determine whether this is a concomitant nonparalytic squint or a noncomitant (paralytic) squint. Paralytic squint results from paralysis of one or more ocular muscles commonly due to lesions of the 3rd, 4th or 6th cranial nerves and is characterized by limitation of eye movement and increasing diplopia in the field of action of the paralysed muscles. In concomitant squint there is muscle imbalance, but the ocular movements are full and the squint may be convergent or divergent.

Common questions

Q. What are the various muscle actions on the eyeball?

A.
Muscle	Nerve supply	Action
Ext. rectus	6th nerve	Abduction
Int. rectus	3rd nerve	Adduction
Sup. oblique	4th nerve	Depression when eye turned inwards
Inf. oblique	3rd nerve	Elevation when eye turned inwards
Sup. rectus	3rd nerve	Elevation when eye turned outwards
Inf. rectus	3rd nerve	Depression when eye turned outwards

Q. What is the commonest cause for a concomitant squint?
A. An uncorrected error of refraction in early childhood is usually the cause for such squints.

58. Nystagmus

You may be asked to examine the eyes. As soon as you check the movements of the eyeballs, involuntary rhythmic oscillations of the eyes should give you this diagnosis. Remember to hold your examining finger at least two feet away from the patient and do not go laterally beyond the range of binocular vision. If the testing finger is held close to the patient's eyes a slight transient nystagmus is often seen and is not pathological.

- Determine whether the nystagmus is pendular (the oscillations are equal in speed and amplitude in both directions) or jerking with quick and slow phases of unequal direction. The quicker phase is arbitrarily used to define the direction of nystagmus.
- If the nystagmus is pendular check the visual acuity and look for features of conditions commonly responsible for this type of nystagmus, e.g. albinism and diseases of the retina causing poor vision (examination of the fundus).
- For the much commoner jerky nystagmus determine whether the nystagmus is horizontal or vertical. Vertical nystagmus usually is a sign of brain stem disease. In vestibular lesions (check for deafness and look at both ears) the slow phase of the nystagmus is towards the diseased side. Acoustic neuroma commonly causes horizontal nystagmus. Also phasic nystagmus is commonly seen in alcoholism and barbiturate poisoning. If a cerebellar lesion is suspected look for other cerebellar signs, e.g. intention tremor, scanning speech, dysdiadochokenesia and hypotonia of the limbs.

Common question

Q. What is a dissociated or ataxic nystagmus?

A. When the nystagmus is seen in the abducted eye only it is called dissociated or ataxic nystagmus and if bilaterally present it is considered to be pathognomic of multiple sclerosis.

59. Horner's syndrome

Locally

You may be asked to look at the face or the eyes.

- Note the partial ptosis on either side.
- Note the small size of the pupil on the same side which fails to respond to the light reflex.
- Look carefully for the small and rather sunken eyeball (enophthalmos).
- Lack of sweating on that side of the face is rather difficult to demonstrate and not considered a very important part of the syndrome.

Elsewhere

Look for any signs of brain stem lesion, e.g. nystagmus.

- Examine the neck for cervical ribs, lymphadenopathy or a scar of injury or operation.
- Check for patchy loss of sensations in the upper limbs (syringomyelia).

Common question

Q. What are the causes of Horner's syndrome?
A. (i) Lesion of the brain stem paralysing the autonomic pathways.
   (ii) C_8–T_1 lesions, e.g. syringomyelia.
   (iii) Lesion in the superior mediastinum, e.g. aneurysm, glandular enlargement, bronchial carcinoma.
   (iv) Lesions in the neck, e.g. trauma, lymphadenopathy.

60. Ptosis

You may be asked to look at the face.

- Note the drooping of the upper eyelids.
- Determine whether the ptosis is unilateral or bilateral, partial

or complete, with or without over-action of the frontalis muscle.

• Look for size of the pupil, light and accommodation reflexes and presence of strabismus (3rd nerve palsy or Horner's syndrome).

• Look for any evidence of myopathy and other features of dystrophia myotonica, e.g. cataract, gonadal atrophy and frontal baldness.

Common question

Q. What are the causes of ptosis?

A. (i) 3rd nerve palsy – ptosis is usually complete, unilateral and with over-action of the frontalis. Paralytic squint with a dilated pupil are additional features.

(ii) Sympathetic paralysis (Horner's syndrome). The ptosis is always partial with small pupil. Remember, and look for, various causes of Horner's syndrome (see Case 59).

(iii) Tabes dorsalis – ptosis is usually bilateral with over-action of the frontalis.

(iv) Myopathies like facioscapulohumeral myopathy, dystrophia myotonica or myasthenia gravis.

(v) Congenital – a common cause of bilateral or unilateral partial ptosis with over-action of frontalis.

(vi) Hysterical ptosis – very rare and is always unilateral.

61. AR (Argyll Robertson) pupils

Locally

• Carefully look at the small, irregular and unequal pupils.

• Check the accommodation and light reflexes. The accommodation reflex is present whereas the pupils do not react to light, both direct and consensual.

• Look for ptosis which usually accompanies.

Elsewhere

• Look for valvular lesion such as aortic incompetence which is syphilitic in origin.

- Check for loss of proprioception with positive Rhomberg's sign.

Common questions

Q. Where is the lesion in this condition?
A. It is not known exactly, but probably in the ciliary ganglion.

Q. What is a Holmes Adie pupil?
A. A condition confined to women, always unilateral and associated with diminished or absent tendon jerks. The pupil is larger than normal with absent light reflex and very slow accommodation reflex.

Q. What are four important characteristics of AR pupils?
A. (i) Bilateral, small, irregular and unequal pupils.
(ii) Pupils fail to dilate properly in response to mydriatric drugs.
(iii) Pupils fail to react to light but accommodation reflex is retained.
(iv) There may be associated atrophy and depigmentation of the iris.

Q. Name four other conditions which may cause AR pupils.
A. Most but not all features of AR pupils may be seen in the following conditions:
(i) Diabetes mellitus.
(ii) Orbital injury.
(iii) Hereditary neuropathies.
(iv) Sarcoidosis.

62. Homonymous hemianopia

You may be asked to check the field of vision of a given patient.

- Sit at about a half-metre distance, opposite the patient.
- Keep your eyes at the same level as those of the patient.
- Test the field of vision separately in each eye and in every direction.

- To localize the lesion check the light reflex as well. If absent the lesion is between the optic chiasma and the mid-brain but if the light reflex is present the lesion is placed between the mid-brain and the occipital lobe.

Discussion

Lesions in the optic tract, optic radiations or cerebral cortex produce homonymous hemianopia, with loss of function in the right or left halves of both visual fields opposite to the side affected. Commonly presented cases are usually with strokes. Bitemporal hemianopia results from pituitary and suprasellar tumours. Just like hemianopia the candidate should also be familiar with scotomas. A scotoma is an area of absent or partial loss of vision within the visual field. A lesion of the optic nerve causes central scotoma, as commonly seen in multiple sclerosis.

63. Central scotoma

You may be asked to examine the field of vision of a patient who has central scotoma.

- Examine the field of vision by asking the patient to sit upright, directly facing you approximately two feet away. For testing his right eye, ask the patient to cover his left eye, your own right eye being closed. You should be looking steadily in the patient's right eye with your left eye. Use a pin with a large head (hat pin). Check the peripheral extent of the fields by bringing the pin into the field of vision from the periphery at several points on the circumference. Examine from all quadrants so as to be sure about the complete field of vision on that side.
- Now similarly examine for the left eye.
- Note for any loss of field of vision in the centre and this is called central scotoma.
- Once you have decided about the presence of central scotoma, look into the fundus with your ophthalmoscope for any temporal pallor of the disc and other evidence of optic atrophy.

Common question

Q. What are the common causes of central scotoma?

A. (i) Retrobulbar neuritis, most commonly in cases of multiple sclerosis.

(ii) Optic atrophy due to toxins or B_{12} deficiency.

(iii) Pressure on the optic nerve by a tumour.

(iv) Choroidoretinitis.

Looking at the Fundi

64. Papilloedema

You may be asked to look at the fundus and in a short case it should suffice if you can recognize the presence of papilloedema. Remember, and look for, the different stages of papilloedema and these are:

- Engorgement of the retinal veins.
- Blurring of the disc margins.
- A redder disc with loss of physiological cupping of the disc.

Common questions

Q. What are the causes of papilloedema?
A. (i) Raised intracranial pressure.
   (ii) Malignant hypertension.
   (iii) Central retinal vein thrombosis.
   (iv) Optic neuritis/papillitis.
   (v) Rarely, hypercapnia; hypoparathyroidism.

Q. How is papillitis different from papilloedema?
A. In papillitis, the condition is usually unilateral with loss of visual acuity, whereas in papilloedema the condition is usually bilateral and the visual acuity remains normal, but there is an enlargement of the blind spot.

Q. What is Foster Kennedy syndrome?
A. Papilloedema on one side and optic atrophy on the other is

called Foster Kennedy syndrome. This may be caused by a tumour of the frontal lobe, which may cause optic atrophy because of the pressure on the optic nerve. With increase in the size of the tumour there is a rise in the intracranial pressure, and this causes papilloedema on the other side.

65. Optic atrophy

You may be asked to examine the fundus.

- Note the pallor of the disc. A pale disc signifies optic atrophy.
- Look for any evidence of papilloedema, disc contour, cup and cribrosa.
- Look at the vessels and see if the veins and arterioles are normal or attenuated.

Common questions

Q. How do you differentiate primary from the secondary optic atrophy?

A.

Primary	*Secondary*
No preceding papilloedema	Definite preceding papilloedema
Disc contour, cup and cribrosa well circumscribed	They are ill-defined
Veins and arterioles are attenuated	Arteries attenuated, veins remain congested
Causes Multiple sclerosis Tabes dorsalis B12 deficiency Diabetes mellitus Toxic – tobacco, methyl alcohol Familial cerebellar ataxia	Causes Brain tumour Temporal arteritis Thrombosis of central retinal artery

Q. What is consecutive optic atrophy?
A. Optic atrophy due to a disease within the eye causing optic

nerve damage (glaucoma, choroiditis, retinitis pigmentosa) is sometimes termed 'consecutive optic atrophy'. Some people include consecutive optic atrophy as a part of secondary optic atrophy.

66. Diabetic fundus

You may be asked to look at the fundus of a diabetic patient. The changes may be of background retinopathy as described below:

* Microaneurysms with tortuous and congested veins.
* Haemorrhages which are in the form of dots and blots.
* Exudates which are usually 'hard' and waxy with well defined edges.

In addition to background retinopathy the following features of proliferative retinopathy must be looked for:

* Neovascularization, i.e. new vessel formation over the disc and along the nerves. Macular oedema may also accompany.
* Pre-retinal haemorrhages.
* Subhyaloid haemorrhages. Boat-shaped vitreous haemorrhages.
* Retinal detachment.

Common question

Q. What is the treatment for proliferative retinopathy?
A. Photocoagulation.
   Pituitary ablation.

67. Hypertensive fundus

You may be asked to look into the fundus of a hypertensive patient. Note and describe the retinal changes of various grades:

* *Grade I*   Irregularity of the lumen of the arteriole, with increased light reflex.

- *Grade II*   Arteriovenous nipping.
- *Grade III*   Haemorrhages, most commonly flame-shaped, and exudates.
- *Grade IV*   Papilloedema.

Common questions

Q. Tell me something about the exudates.

A. The soft (cotton wool) exudates are poorly demarcated superficial ischaemic areas of the necrosis of the retina, or localized collections of oedema fluid in the nerve fibre layers. These indicate the onset of the accelerated or malignant phase of the hypertension and commonly disappear within a few weeks with good control of hypertension. Hard exudates are small, deep, dense deposits of lipids and have well defined borders. They persist much longer than the soft exudates.

Q. What are the important causes of exudates?

A. (i) Hypertension.
   (ii) Diabetes mellitus.
   (iii) Systemic lupus erythematosus (cytoid bodies).
   (iv) Severe anaemia.
   (v) Leukaemia.

68. Choroiditis

You may be asked to look at the fundus.

- Carefully note the exudates appearing as white opaque areas of varying sizes, surrounded by a black pigmented margin.
- Note that the retinal vessels are always superficial to the exudates.

Common questions

Q. What are the causes of choroiditis?

A. (i) Toxoplasmosis.
   (ii) Sarcoidosis.
   (iii) Tuberculosis.

(iv) Syphilis.
(v) Trauma.

Q. What four investigations would you ask for?
A. (i) CXR.
   (ii) Sabin–Feldman dye test (high titres of antibody).
   (iii) Serological test for syphilis.
   (iv) Kveim test for sarcoidosis.

69. Retinitis pigmentosa

You may be asked to look at the fundus.

- Note the exudates as described for choroiditis. But the essential difference is that the exudates in retinitis pigmentosa interrupt the vessels since the exudates are much more superficial.
- Look for any evidence of secondary optic atrophy.
- Check the visual field for 'tunnel vision' (constricted visual fields).
- Check for any motor and sensory neuropathy and ataxia since presence of such features would point towards the diagnosis of Refsum's disease. Much more commonly the patient may have Laurence–Moon–Biedl syndrome (see Case 20).

Common questions

Q. What is the inheritance of this condition?
A. Retinitis pigmentosa is inherited as an autosomal recessive disorder. In some cases it may be autosomal dominant or, rarely, sex-linked.

Q. What is the treatment of this condition?
A. No effective therapy is available yet. Most patients are registered blind and thus eligible for benefits and aids.

70. Embolism (occlusion) of the central artery of the retina

- Look at the macular region for a peculiar round 'cherry red' spot (bright red spot on the fovea).

- Note that the arteries are attenuated and there may be streaky haemorrhages around the vessels.
- Note that the veins are narrow too, with less blood than normal.
- The optic disc is pale and atrophied (see Case 65).
- Check for visual acuity (vision is completely lost as a result of sudden complete blindness in the affected eye).

Common question

Q. What are the causes of such an occlusion?
A. (i) Cranial arteritis.
   (ii) Embolus from infective endocarditis.
   (iii) Disseminated atherosclerotic plaque.

71. Retinal vein thrombosis

You may be asked to look at the fundus.

- Note the papilloedema and oedema of the rest of the retina which is usually unilateral.
- Note gross venous distension and numerous haemorrhages.
- Test for the visual acuity which is affected.
- Look for the presence of microaneurysms or collateral vessels which may be present.

Common questions

Q. How do you differentiate this condition from papilloedema?
A. Papilloedema is usually bilateral whereas retinal vein thrombosis is unilateral. Moreover the visual acuity in papilloedema usually remains normal until the late stages whereas it is affected at an early stage in retinal vein thrombosis.

Q. What are the causes of retinal vein thrombosis?
A. (i) Hyperviscosity syndrome (myeloma, myeloproliferative disorders).
   (ii) Hypertension.
   (iii) Diabetes mellitus.

Looking at the Hands

72. Hands with joint swelling

You may be asked to look at the hands. Commonly given cases are those of rheumatoid arthritis, psoriasis, osteoarthritis and gout and you must remember the important differentiating features of these conditions.

Locally

- Note the swelling with or without ulnar deviation of the meta-carpophalangeal (MCP) joints.
- Note that only the proximal interphalangeal joints (not the distal ones) are involved in rheumatoid arthritis.
- Since the patient could have both rheumatoid and osteoarthritis, look for the presence of Heberden's nodes at the terminal interphalangeal joints.
- Look for Swan neck deformity or trigger finger (tendon sheath involvement) and Boutonnière (button hole) deformity.
- Any associated palmar erythema?
- Look for pitting of the nails to exclude psoriasis. Remember that psoriatic arthropathy is seronegative and characteristically involves the terminal interphalangeal joints with absence of subcutaneous nodules.
- Look for lumpy swellings (tophi) of the joints, sometimes seen with superficial ulceration and chalky material through the shiny skin.

Elsewhere

• Look for rheumatoid nodules, if present, around the elbow joints on the extensor surface.
• Look for tophi in the cartilage of the ears.
• Also check for evidence of arthropathy in other joints like knees and elbows.
• Check for vasculitis lesions in the nail folds (rheumatoid arthritis) or pitting of the nails (psoriasis).
• Look for psoriatic lesions on the skin, most commonly on the extensor aspects.

Common question

Q. What two investigations would you ask for?
A. (i) X-ray of both hands.
   (ii) Latex rheumatoid factor.

73. Small muscle atrophy of the hands

Locally

• Look for the wasting of the small muscles including thenar and hypothenar eminences.
• Test the various muscles supplied by median and ulnar nerves in the hand (see Cases 85, 86, 87) including the reflexes in the upper limbs.
• Test for any sensory deficit/fasciculations.
• Look carefully for any evidence of rheumatoid arthritis, e.g. swelling of MCP joints with ulnar deviation.

Elsewhere

• Always examine the other hand as discussed above.
• Look behind the elbows for evidence of possible trauma to the ulnar nerve.
• Look for features of Horner's syndrome (ptosis, miosis and enophthalmos).

- Examine the neck for any operation scar, cervical ribs etc.
- Look for pyramidal signs in the lower limbs.

Common conditions

- Rheumatoid arthritis.
- Peripheral nerve lesion, e.g. median and ulnar nerves.
- In the spinal cord (intramedullary), e.g. motor neurone disease, syringomyelia, tumours.
- Outside the spinal cord (extramedullary), e.g. cervical spondylosis, cervical rib, tumours.

Discussion

There are many causes of small muscle atrophy of the hand which may or may not be symmetrical in both hands. In motor neurone disease the reflexes in the upper limbs are usually brisk and not lost unless the muscles are grossly paralysed. Fasciculation is common and there is no sensory loss. In amyotrophic lateral sclerosis pyramidal signs are present in the lower limbs. In syringomyelia besides wasting there is patchy loss of pain and temperature sensation in both arms and sometimes there may be signs of Horner's syndrome on either side. Spinal cord tumours are characterized by wasting, sensory disturbance and absent tendon reflexes in the upper limbs. With pancoast tumour and cervical rib sensory loss in the ulnar nerve distribution commonly accompanies wasting of the small muscles. Wasting in the cases of carpal tunnel syndrome, median and ulnar nerve lesions has been discussed elsewhere (Cases 83, 87 and 84 respectively).

74. Palmar erythema

Locally

- Note the redness of the palms, especially over the thenar, hypothenar eminences and the pulps of the fingers.

Elsewhere

- Since the commonest association is with liver cell disease, look for signs such as Dupuytren's contracture, spider naevi, hepatosplenomegaly, ascites, oedema of the legs, gynaecomastia, absent secondary sexual hair, etc.
- Rarely the soles of the feet may also show redness.

Common conditions

- Cirrhosis of the liver.
- Pregnancy.
- Females on contraceptive pills.
- Thyrotoxicosis.
- Rheumatoid arthritis.
- Some normal people.

Discussion

Palmar erythema is a persistent extensive redness of the palms due to local vasodilatation with increased blood flow. The cardiac output is usually increased in patients with prominent palmar erythema. Skin over the thenar, hypothenar and finger pulp eminences is markedly red as compared to the rest of the palm.

75. Dupuytren's contracture

Locally

- Ask the patient to spread the fingers so as not to miss this condition.
- Also make sure that you examine both hands so as not to miss the condition on the other hand.
- Early Dupuytren's contracture may be easily missed unless the candidate is careful not to forget to palpate the palmar fascia.
- Look for palmar erythema, clubbing and leuconychia.

Elsewhere

- Since the commonest association is with cirrhosis of the liver, look for other stigmata, e.g. spider naevi, hepatospleno-megaly, ascites, oedema of the legs, etc.

Common conditions

- Portal cirrhosis.
- Rheumatoid arthritis.
- Familial.
- Epileptics.
- Trauma (gardners, vibrating machines).

Discussion

The fibrosis and thickening of the palmar fascia and of the flexor tendons is the underlying pathology. This subsequently results in the flexion deformity of their metacarpophalangeal joints, especially of the ring and the middle fingers and loss of function of the fingers. It is important to palpate the palm so as not to miss the thickened fascia in cases of early Dupuytren's contracture. In most cases the condition becomes bilateral. Further the condition should be carefully differentiated from ulnar nerve palsy where the dorsal and palmar interossei muscles are paralysed with resultant loss of flexion of proximal phalanx, extension of dorsal phalanx, adduction and abduction of fingers. Also there would be loss of sensation over the ulnar border of the hand (see Case 85).

76. Clubbing of the fingers

Locally

- Make sure this is significant clubbing with the thickened tissue at the base of the nail with obliteration of the angle between the base of the nail and the adjacent skin of the finger.
- Note the convexity of the nail from above down as well as from side to side.

- Look for the 'drumstick' appearance of the fingers.
- Check for presence of abnormal flucuation at the nail bases.
- Check for any evidence of hypertrophic pulmonary osteo-arthropathy and painful swelling of the ends of radius and ulna due to periosteal thickening.

Elsewhere

- Look for dyspnoea and cyanosis.
- Examine the chest for conditions like bronchiectasis, lung abscess, carcinoma and fibrosing alveolitis.
- Examine the cardiovascular system for any evidence of congenital heart disease.

Common question

Q. What are the causes of clubbing?
A. (i) Respiration system, e.g. bronchiectasis, lung abscess, carcinoma of the lung, fibrosing alveolitis.
(ii) Cardiovascular system, e.g. cyanotic heart disease, infective endocarditis, atrial myxoma.
(iii) Liver and GI tract, e.g. Crohn's disease, ulcerative colitis, coeliac disease, primary biliary cirrhosis of the liver.
(iv) Familial/idiopathic clubbing.
(v) Thyrotoxicosis (thyroid acropachy).

77. Splinter haemorrhage

Locally

- Look very carefully so as not to miss these lesions.
- Look at the nails of the fingers on the other hand as well.

Elsewhere

- Look for other features of conditions like infective endo-carditis, e.g. petechial haemorrhages (in conjunctiva or oral mucosa, anaemia, splenomegaly, Osler's nodes, Roth spots, Janeway lesions, etc.

Common conditions

- Trauma, especially in manual labourers.
- Infective endocarditis.
- Septicaemia.

Discussion

Haemorrhages in the nail beds usually have a linear distribution near the distal end, hence the name 'splinter haemorrhages'. Remember these haemorrhages are not considered to be pathognomonic of infective endocarditis. They are thought to be caused by dissemination of tiny thrombi. Do not forget the differentiation of splinter haemorrhages from trichiniasis (very rare in the UK). Splinter haemorrhages are longitudinal whereas in trichiniasis the haemorrhages are always transverse.

78. Leuconychia

Locally

- Look carefully for the whiteness of the whole nail, or bands or flecks of whiteness.

Elsewhere

- Look for various stigmata of liver cell disease (cirrhosis), as discussed in Case 44.

Discussion

Hypoalbuminaemia due to any cause may cause leuconychia. Cirrhosis of the liver, nephrotic syndrome, protein-losing enteropathy and chronic inorganic arsenic poisoning are important causes. Do remember that small isolated white patches may sometimes be seen in the nails of normal persons.

Common question

Q. What two investigations would you ask for?
A. (i) Liver function tests.
   (ii) Urine examination (proteinuria).

79. Marfan's syndrome

You may be asked to look at the hands.

Locally

- Look carefully at the long spider like fingers (arachnodactyly).
- Patient is taller than average – with an arm span greater than his height.

Elsewhere

- Check for hyperextensibility of joints, flat feet and kypho-scoliosis.
- In the eyes – subluxation of the lens and iridodonesis.
- Look for high arched palate.
- Cardiovascular changes – aortic or mitral regurgitation.

Discussion

Marfan's syndrome is an inherited disorder of an unknown element of connective tissue, resulting in ocular, skeletal and cardiovascular abnormalities. It is transmitted as an autosomal dominant trait. There is a wide variability in clinical severity. Homocystinuria is frequently confused with Marfan's syndrome because of similar skeletal, ocular and cardiovascular abnormalities but can be differentiated by downwards lens dislocation (upward in Marfan's syndrome) and mental retardation (70% of cases) and by finding homocystine in the urine.

80. Syringomyelia/syringobulbia

You may be asked to look at the hands.

- Note the wasting of the small muscles of the hands with or without trophic lesions.
- Check for segmental areas of loss of pain and temperature sensation and see if there is any scar of painless burn or cut on the fingers.
- Look for signs of lower motor neurone lesions in the upper limbs (due to the involvement of the anterior horn cells) and upper motor neurone lesions in the lower limbs due to involvement of the pyramidal tracts.
- Look for signs of Horner's syndrome on either side (see Case 59).
- Look for the presence of nystagmus (probably due to involvement of fibres of the vestibulospinal tracts.)
- Look for fasciculations.

Common question

Q. What is the treatment for this condition?
A. Rather unsatisfactory; surgery is sometimes helpful.

81. Heberden's nodes

Locally

- Heberden's nodes are osteophytes at the distal interphalangeal joints.
- Look for similar bony swellings at the proximal interphalangeal joints (Bouchard's nodes) and metacarpophalangeal joints, specially the first (thumb) metacarpophalangeal joint.
- Note that the patient is usually obese and elderly.

Elsewhere

- Look for the evidence of osteoarthritis in other joints, especially the knees and the hips.

Common question

Q. What single investigation would you ask for?
A. X-ray hands.

82. Swelling of the phalanges

Locally

- Note that the swelling is in the phalanges and not in the joints.
- Look at the other hand as well for similar involvement of the phalanges.

Elsewhere

- Look at the face for any evidence of lupus pernio, a bluish discoloration on the nose, not uncommonly seen in cases of sarcoidosis.
- Also look for any evidence of uveitis.

Common conditions

- Sarcoidosis.
- Sickle cell disease.
- Chronic infection of the bone (rare).

Common question

Q. What two investigations could you ask for?
A. (i) X-ray of chest and hands.
   (ii) Kveim test.

83. Carpal tunnel syndrome

You may be asked to examine the hand of a patient whose main complaint may be the painful tingling of the hands.

Locally

- Look for any scar of injury or bony deformity which might suggest previous trauma to the wrist joint.
- Look at both hands carefully for any evidence of rheumatoid arthritis or wasting of small muscles of the hands – for example, of the outer part of the thenar eminence in the above syndrome. If present, then test the muscles of the thumb, e.g. opponens and abductor pollicis brevis (supplied by median nerve) and note their weakness.
- Now examine for any sensory loss over the palmar aspects of the thumb, index finger, middle and radial half of the ring fingers (the rest of the palm being normal).
- Ask for any paraesthesiae experienced by the patient on percussion over the carpal ligament (Tinel's sign).

Elsewhere

- Look carefully for any features of acromegaly, hypothyroidism and amyloidosis.

Common question

Q. What are the common causes of this syndrome?
A. (i) Local trauma.
   (ii) Rheumatoid arthritis.
   (iii) Acromegaly.
   (iv) Hypothyroidism.
   (v) Pregnancy.
   (vi) Premenstrual oedema.

84. Absent radial pulse (either side)

Locally

- Once again it is important to check both radial pulses simultaneously, to assess whether there is any gross difference between the two sides.
- If on one side the radial is feeble or completely missing, feel for

brachial, axillary and subclavian arteries, respectively.
- Listen for any bruit (carotid/vertebral) on either side of the neck.
- Look for any mass compressing the arteries in the neck.

Common conditions

- Thrombosis/embolism in a peripheral artery.
- Rarely, subclavian artery stenosis.
- Brachial artery catheter.

Common questions

Q. How is the circle of Willis formed?

A. Anterior, middle and posterior cerebral arteries joined through anterior and posterior communicating arteries form the circle of Willis.

Q. What is pulseless (Takayasu's) disease?

A. It is a rare condition occurring particularly in young women, first described by Takayasu in Japan. All three major trunks arising from the aortic arch are affected, resulting in coronary insufficiency, absent pulses in the arms and symptoms of cerebral ischaemia.

Q. What is subclavian steal syndrome?

A. It is a rare condition in which symptoms of vertebrobasilar insufficiency are experienced by the patient on exercising his arm, since the subclavian artery distal to the stenosis 'steals' blood retrogradely from the vertebral artery. The condition is seen in cases of subclavian artery stenosis, at or near its origin.

85. Claw hands (ulnar nerve palsy)

Locally

- Note that the proximal (metacarpophalangeal joints) phalanges are over-extended and the interphalangeal joints are flexed, with slight separation of the ring and little fingers, and with wasting of small muscles.

- Remember to test all the muscles in the forearm and various small muscles of the hand supplied by ulnar nerve.
- Test for any loss of cutaneous sensation supplied by the ulnar nerve ($C_8 T_1$), e.g. ulnar border of the hand both on dorsal and palmar aspects, little finger and the ulnar half of the ring finger.

Elsewhere

- Always examine both hands.
- Look around the olecranon groove and the wrist for any visible scar or fracture as evidence of possible injury to the ulnar nerve.
- If both hands are affected, the lesion is likely to be more central, i.e. at $C_8 T_1$ level, such as syringomyelia, motor neurone disease, cervical spondylosis and cervical cord tumours.

Discussion

The interossei adduct and abduct the fingers and, if the power of the long flexors and extensors of the fingers is retained and the interossei are paralysed, the so called claw hand or main-engriffe deformity is seen. The candidate is advised to remember and practice testing all the muscles supplied by ulnar nerve, as summarized below.

Cord segments	Muscles supplied	Action to be tested
$C_{7,8}, T_1$	Flexor carpi ulnaris	Ulnar flexion of hand
$C_{7,8}, T_1$	Flexor digitorum profundus (medial half)	Flexion of terminal phalanx of ring and little fingers against resistance
C_8, T_1	Adductor pollicis	Adduction of metacarpal of thumb, by asking patient to attempt to hold a piece of paper between the thumb and palmar aspect of the forefinger

Cord segments	Muscle supplied	Action to be tested
C_8, T_1	Abductor digiti minimi	Abduction of little finger
$C_{7,8}$, T_1	Opponens digiti minimi	Opposition of little finger
$C_{7,8}$, T_1	Flexor digiti minimi	Flexion of little finger
C_8, T_1	Dorsal and palmar interossei and lumbricals III and IV	Flexion of proximal phalanx, extension of two distal phalanges, and adduction and abduction of fingers

86. Wrist drop

You may be asked to look at the hand of a patient with radial nerve injury.

- Note that the patient is unable to extend the wrist, the fingers at the metacarpophalangeal joints, and the thumb.
- Look for any scar of injury, especially in the spiral groove on the shaft of the humerus.
- Look for any area of sensory loss, especially on the posterior aspect of the thumb and on the dorsoradial side of the hand. If the nerve is damaged higher up, above the origin of the posterior cutaneous nerve, a strip along the posterior surface of the forearm may show loss of sensation.
- Remember the cord segments, muscles supplied and their actions, as given below.

Cord segments	Muscles supplied	Action to be tested
C_{6-8}	Triceps and anconeus	Extension of forearm
$C_{5,6}$	Brachioradialis	Flexion of forearm
C_{5-7}	Extensor carpiradialis	Radial extension of hand
C_{6-8}	Extensor digitorum	Extension of phalanges of all four fingers in the hand
C_{6-8}	Extensor digiti minimi	Extension of phalanges of little finger

Cord segments	Muscle supplied	Action to be tested
C_{6-8}	Extensor carpi ulnaris	Ulnar extension of hand
C_{5-7}	Supinator	Supination of forearm
$C_{6,7}$	Abductor pollicis longus	Abduction of metacarpal of thumb
$C_{6,7}$	Extensor pollicis brevis	Extension of thumb
C_{6-8}	Extensor digitorum longus	Extension of index finger

87. Median nerve palsy

You may be asked to look at a hand with median nerve damage.

- Look for any scar of injury around the wrist.
- Note the wastings of the thenar eminence, and the thumb falling in a flat ape-like position.
- Test for loss of sensation in the volar aspect of the thumb, index and middle fingers.
- Remember to test for the muscle functions supplied by the median nerve, as given below

Cord segments	Muscles supplied	Action to be tested
$C_{6,7}$	Pronator teres	Pronation of forearm
$C_{6,7}$	Flexor carpi radialis	Radial flexion of hand
$C_{7,8},\ T_1$	Palmaris longus	Flexion of hand
$C_{7,8},\ T_1$	Flexor digitorum superficialis	Flexion of middle phalanx of all four fingers
$C_{6,7}$	Flexor pollicis longus	Flexion of terminal phalanx of thumb
$C_{7,8},\ T_1$	Flexor digitorum profundus	Flexion of terminal phalanx of index and middle fingers
$C_{6,7}$	Abductor pollicis brevis	Abduction of metacarpal of thumb

Cord segments	Muscles supplied	Action to be tested
$C_{6,7}$	Flexor pollicis brevis	Flexion of proximal phalanx of thumb
$C_{6,7}$	Opponens pollicis	Opposition of metacarpal of thumb
C_8, T_1	Two lateral lumbricals	Flexion of proximal phalanx and extension of the two distal phalanges of index and middle fingers

88. Intention tremor

You may be asked to examine the upper limbs and during the course of your examination you may notice the ataxia which appear during movement of a limb and disappear at rest. These ataxic movements are called intention tremor.

- Look for other signs of cerebellar disease, e.g. finger to nose test for ataxia, scanning speech or dysarthria, nystagmus and hypotonia.
- Since patients with multiple sclerosis are commonly presented as short cases, the candidate may look for upgoing plantar reflexes with spasticity of lower limbs (with the permission of the examiner).

Common question

Q. What is a tic?
A. Tics are repetitive purposive acts which are first started voluntarily but later become involuntary and habitual. Blinking of the eyes, nodding of the head or smacking of the lips are common examples.

Looking at the Legs

89. Bowing of the legs (Paget's disease)

Locally

- Note the lateral bowing of the legs.
- Palpate and feel whether the local temperature of the affected area over the bone is raised due to increased vascularity and arteriovenous fistula. The subcutaneous surface of the tibia is often widened. Also occasionally a bruit may be audible locally.
- Look for any oedema of the legs – a part of the congestive cardiac failure associated with Paget's disease of the bone.

Elsewhere

- Look at the skull for enlarged calvarium, since the skull is commonly affected.
- Look for deformities of the other bones if present, e.g. pelvis, humerus, spine, clavicle, etc.
- Look for signs of high output cardiac failure, e.g. a collapsing pulse, raised JVP, cardiomegaly, hepatomegaly and oedema of the legs as mentioned earlier.
- Check for deafness.

Common conditions

- Paget's disease of the bone.

- Rickets or osteomalacia.
- Sabre tibia where the bowing of the legs is anteriorly, and is due to congenital syphilis.

Discussion

Paget's disease of the bone is seldom seen before the age of 50 years and its aetiology remains unknown. There is evidence of both increased osteoblastic and osteoclastic activity.

Common questions

Q. What two important investigations should you do?
A. (i) X-ray of the bones.
   (ii) Serum alkaline phosphatase.

Q. What are the complications of Paget's disease?
A. (i) Bone pains.
   (ii) Pathological fractures.
   (iii) Congestive cardiac failure.
   (iv) Osteogenic sarcoma.
   (v) Cranial nerve palsy – most commonly of the 8th nerve.

Q. Discuss the differential diagnosis of three major causes of bowing legs.
A.

Paget's disease	Rickets	Sabre tibia (congenital syphilis)
Patient is usually of normal height but with a stoop	Patient is usually of short stature	Patient is usually a dwarf
Skull commonly involved, with enlarged calvarium with an irregular surface. Also, deafness may be present due to 8th nerve involvement	Bossing of frontal and parietal bones	Bossing of frontal and parietal bones; a depressed bridge of nose due to 'snuffles' may be seen

Paget's disease	Rickets	Sabre tibia (congenital syphilis)
Pelvis, humerus, clavicle, tibia and femur may be involved	Pelvic deformities may be seen. In the chest: 'rickety rosary', pigeon chest, funnel chest, Harrison's sulcus and kypho-scoliosis may be seen	Other stigmata of congenital syphilis, e.g. interstitial kera-titis, corneal opacity, choroiditis, optic atrophy, Hutchinsons' incisors (notched and peg-shaped teeth) may be present
Bowing of the legs with rise in temperature over the legs due to increased vascularity	Bowing of both legs but no evidence of increased vascularity	Sabre tibia may be unilateral and the bowing is anteriorly and not laterally
There may be evidence of high output cardiac failure	No evidence of high output cardiac failure	No evidence of high output cardiac failure
Biochemical findings		
	(active rickets)	
Calcium – normal	– normal or low	– normal
Phosphorus – normal	– low	– normal
Alkaline phosphatase – raised	– raised	– normal

90. Swelling of one leg

Locally

- Determine whether the oedema is pitting or non-pitting.
- Compare skin colour with other leg.
- Determine whether the local temperature of the skin is raised or not.
- Look for a positive Homan's sign.
- Measure the girth of both legs.

Elsewhere

- Check for any lymphadenopathy in the groins.

- Look for any abdominal mass causing obstruction to the venous flow of the leg.
- Examine knee joint.

Common conditions

- Deep vein thrombosis of the leg.
- Cellulitis of the leg.
- Lymphoedema.
- Ruptured Baker's cyst.

Discussion

Thrombosis in the deep veins of the leg is a common condition and always carries a risk of pulmonary embolism. Over half the patients with deep vein thrombosis have no physical signs. Damage to the vessel wall, reduced blood flow and increased coagulability of the blood are important causes to be considered.

91. Swelling of both legs

Locally

- Determine whether the oedema is pitting (venous) or non-pitting (lymphatic), but do remember that venous oedema, if it is chronic enough, becomes non-pitting.
- Determine whether the local temperature of the overlying skin is raised or not.
- Look for varicose veins.
- Measure the girth of both legs.
- Look for lymphadenopathy in the groins.
- Remember that most patients are obese middle-aged females if the swelling is due to primary lymphoedema.

Elsewhere

- Look for raised JVP, hepatomegaly, heart murmurs and congestion of the lungs (basal crepitations), since congestive cardiac failure is probably the commonest cause of bilateral pitting oedema of the legs.

- Hypoalbuminaemia due to nephrotic syndrome or cirrhosis of the liver can also cause bilateral pitting of the legs, so look for important and relevant clinical signs, e.g. renal enlargement, puffiness over the eyelids (nephrotic syndrome) or stigmata of cirrhosis such as hepatosplenomegaly, ascites, spider naevi, palmar erythema, Dupuytren's contracture, etc.

Discussion

Primary lymphoedema (Milroy's disease) affects females predominantly, and the onset of the disease occurs before the age of 40 years in most cases. Filariasis in the tropics commonly causes lymphoedema. Neoplastic infiltration of the lymph nodes or the surgical removal of the lymph nodes are other more common causes.

92. Gangrene of the toes

You may be asked to look at the foot of a patient with gangrene, of one or more toes, or a part of the foot.

- Note the area of black discoloration over the toe or part of the foot.
- The area proximal to the gangrene may show atrophic changes – pale, cold and shiny with the presence of superficial ulcers.
- Palpate the peripheral arteries (dorsalis pedis, posterior tibial, popliteal and femoral) for arterial insufficiency both on the side of the gangrene and the other leg.
- If the femoral or popliteal artery is not palpable, auscultate for a systolic bruit over that artery and listen to determine whether or not the pulsations are present.
- Now examine the lower limbs for any evidence of peripheral neuropathy, since in cases of diabetes mellitus, the two conditions commonly coexist.

Common questions

Q. What single investigation would you like to do?
A. Examination of urine for sugar.

Q. What are three common causes of gangrene of the toes?
A. (i) Diabetes mellitus.
   (ii) Arterial embolism.
   (iii) Thrombo-angiitis obliterans (Buerger's disease).

93. Leg Ulcer

Locally

- Look for the size, surface and edges of the ulcer.
- Palpate the peripheral arteries for any evidence of peripheral vascular disease.
- Look for the presence of the varicose eczema, with or without varicose veins.

Elsewhere

- Look at the hands for any evidence of arthropathy.
- Look at the face for the presence of xanthelasma.
- Look for any evidence of splenomegaly.

Common conditions

The following are the commonly seen ulcers on the legs.

(a) Varicose ulcers
Venous incompetency causing increasing oedema, eczema and secondary bacterial infection commonly results in varicose ulceration around the ankles – most commonly around internal malleolus, lower and medial aspect of the leg. Remember that the 'eczema' in varicose ulcers is due to brownish haemosiderin pigmentation and not due to an eczematous skin rash.

(b) Ischaemic ulcers
These are commonly seen in the extreme degree of peripheral vascular disease. The limb is usually cold to touch with poor or absent peripheral pulses.

(c) Rheumatoid arthritis
The ulcers are usually over the lower legs and tend to be deep and indolent. There may be areas of vasculitis in the finger tips. Rheumatoid hands, with or without splenomegaly, should be associated features.

(d) Necrobiosis lipoidica diabeticorum
These lesions are yellowish red sclerotic plaques most commonly seen on shins with ulceration.

(e) Pyoderma gangrenosum
The ulcers have elevated purulent border with gross under-mining of the skin and a zone of erythema beyond the edge. These ulcers are commonly seen on the legs but sometimes may involve the trunk. Besides ulcerative colitis, multiple myeloma and leukaemia are other conditions associated with these ulcers.

(f) Sickle cell anaemia
Punched out, sharply marginated round or oval ulcers in a coloured patient should lead the candidate to suspect sickle cell anaemia as a cause of leg ulcers.

(g) Syphilitic ulcers
Occasionally in cases of tertiary syphilis a sloughing gummatous ulcer with punched out edges may be seen most commonly below the knee.

94. Gout

You may be asked to look at the feet.

- Look at the metatarsophalangeal joint of the big toe which will be red, swollen and tender. The big toe is the first joint to be affected in over 85% of gout cases.
- Examine for the swelling and deformity of other joints, e.g. ankles, knees, wrists, elbows, shoulders, hips and hands, as in the chronic form the condition becomes polyarticular.
- Look carefully for the presence of tophi, which consist of deposits of urates in the periarticular tissues and the cartilages of the ears.

Common questions

Q. What are the three investigations you would like to ask for?
A. (i) Full blood count and ESR.
   (ii) Serum uric acid.
   (iii) X-ray of the affected joint.

Q. What are three common precipitating factors for an acute gouty attack?
A. (i) Alcohol.
   (ii) Thiazide diuretics.
   (iii) Trauma.

Q. What are the three most useful drugs for an acute attack?
A. (i) Colchicine.
   (ii) Indomethacin.
   (iii) Phenylbutazone.

Q. What are the three differential diagnoses?
A. (i) Local cellulitis.
   (ii) Simple trauma to the joint.
   (iii) Pyogenic arthritis.

95. Erythema nodosum

You may be asked to look at the legs.

- Note rounded nodules (usually painful) up to 5 cm in diameter on the anterior surface of the legs.
- Look for similar lesions on the extensor surfaces of the arms.
- Look into the throat for any evidence of sore throat and tonsillitis. (Since this usually precedes erythema nodosum by 2–3 weeks, the findings are often normal.)
- Examine the respiratory system for any evidence of tuberculosis or sarcoidosis, commonly causing erythema nodosum.

Common questions

Q. What are the important causes of erythema nodosum?
A. (i) Streptococcal infection.
   (ii) Sarcoidosis.

(iii) Drug sensitivity (sulphonamides, oral contraceptives, aspirin, etc.)
(iv) Tuberculosis.
(v) Rheumatic fever.
(vi) Idiopathic.

Q. What single question would you like to ask the patient?
A. What drugs has the patient been taking recently?

Q. What three investigations would you ask for?
A. (i) CXR.
(ii) ASO (antistreptolysine O) titre.
(iii) Mantoux test.

96. Pes cavus

Locally

● Note the high arched foot.
● Test for any motor or sensory deficit in both lower limbs.

Elsewhere

● Check for features of syringomyelia, e.g. wasting and trophic lesions of the hands with dissociated sensory loss and upper motor neurone signs in the lower limbs.
● Look for features of Friedreich's ataxia, e.g. ataxia, intention tremor, dysarthria and nystagmus (spinocerebellar tract), impaired joint and vibration sensation (posterior column), extensor plantar reflexes (corticospinal tracts) and optic atrophy. Absent ankle jerk with extensor plantar reflexes may be the sole manifestation. In peroneal muscle atrophy the legs look like inverted champagne bottles. (See Case 97 for other features of this condition, since pes cavus may be a feature of Charcot–Marie–Tooth disease.)

Discussion

Increased height of the longitudinal arch commonly associated with dorsal contracture of the metatarsophalangeal joints results in pes cavus. Most commonly it is not associated with other neurological conditions, but association with Friedreich's ataxia, peroneal muscular atrophy, syringomyelia and spina bifida should be kept in mind.

97. Charcot–Marie–Tooth disease

You may be asked to look at the legs.

Locally

- Note the atrophy in the distal aspect of the thigh resulting in so-called 'inverted champagne bottle' shape of the legs.
- Perform complete neurological examination of the lower limbs and note the atrophy of the peronei muscles, small muscles of the feet, long toe extensors and ankle dorsiflexors.
- Tendon reflexes are either diminished or absent in these wasted muscles.
- Sense of touch, pressure and joint position, and vibration sensations are usually mildly affected in the lower limbs.
- Pes cavus is commonly present.

Discussion

Charcot–Marie–Tooth disease is a relatively common hereditary disorder, characterized by weakness and atrophy, primarily of peroneal muscles due to segmental demyelination of peripheral nerves and associated degeneration of axons and anterior horn cells. Usually the condition is inherited as an autosomal dominant trait. Commonly these patients are used for 'long cases' but sometimes they are used for short cases too.

Common question

Q. Who was Charcot?
A. Charcot was a French physician and neurologist in the middle of the last century.

Dermatology

98. Psoriasis

Common skin conditions like psoriasis are commonly 'used' as short cases.

- Note that the lesions are well circumscribed macules, which become covered with fine silvery scales. Lesions commonly occur on the extensor aspects.
- Rub the lesions and allow the scales to drop off and then note the numerous small bleeding points on the dermis.
- Look at the nails for any pitting, brittleness or irregular erosion (onycholysis).
- Sometimes an arthropathy of the terminal interphalangeal joints may be seen as well; if so the nails will always be affected.

Common questions

Q. What are the precipitating factors?
A. (i) Local trauma (Koebner phenomenon).
   (ii) Sunburn.
   (iii) Topical skin medication.
   (iv) Chloroquine therapy.
   (v) Systemic infections.

Q. How do you treat the condition?
A. (i) Tar ointments.
   (ii) Antimetabolites like methotrexate.

(iii) Dithranol ointment.
(iv) Topical steroids.
(v) PUVA.

99. Acanthosis nigricans

This is an uncommon, but interesting, skin condition.

• Note carefully the thickened, dark brown pigmented patch of the skin, usually bilateral and common in the axillae.

• Look for any evidence of underlying malignancy such as carcinoma of stomach, bowel or the lung since such an association is known to exist in more than 50% of cases.

Discussion

Though acanthosis nigricans developing in the adult is significantly associated with malignancy, it may be genetically determined in some patients and may be present at birth or may develop in childhood. In other cases certain endocrine disorders such as acromegaly, Cushings' syndrome, diabetes mellitus and hypothyroidism may rarely be associated. Skin biopsy for histopathological studies are usually necessary for the diagnosis but this fails to indicate the actual cause for the skin condition.

Common question

Q. What are the other cutaneous manifestations of visceral malignancies?
A. (i) Thrombophlebitis migrans.
   (ii) Dermatomyositis.
   (iii) Gynaecomastia.
   (iv) Ichthyosis (acquired).

100. Vitiligo

Vitiligo is characterized by areas of hypopigmentation. These are commonly seen in exposed areas, particularly the face and dorsal aspects of the hands, mouth, eyes, nose, etc. Most cases are idiopathic.

Since there is an increased incidence of vitiligo with certain autoimmune conditions like pernicious anaemia, hyperthyroidism, Addison's disease and diabetes mellitus, look for associated features of these conditions. However vitiligo in most cases is idiopathic and is thought to have an autoimmune basis itself.

Common questions

Q. What immunological investigation would you ask for?
A. Serum antibodies to thyroid, adrenal and parietal cells.

Q. What is the treatment of this condition?
A. No satisfactory therapy is available. Cosmetic creams, protection from sunlight and oral and topical psoralens have been used with satisfactory results in about one-third of the patients.

Index

NOTES

NOTES